M000294037

TOXIC DENTISTRY EXPOSED

The Link between Dentistry and Modern Chronic Diseases

Dr Graeme Munro-Hall BDS. FIAOMT
Dr Lilian Munro-Hall BDS

AUTHORS
Dr Graeme Munro-Hall BDS FIAOMT
Dr Lilian Munro-Hall BDS

PUBLISHERS
Dr Graeme Munro-Hall BDS FIAOMT
Dr Lilian Munro-Hall BDS

EDITOR
Alastair Hall

TYPESETTER
Alastair Hall

The authors can be contacted at the website
www.toxicdentistryexposed.co.uk

The editor/typesetter can be contacted at labasta@yahoo.com

2nd edition

Drs Graeme Munro-Hall and Lilian Munro-Hall have asserted their right to
be identified as the authors of this work under the Copyright, Designs and
Patents Act 1988.

All rights reserved. No part of this publication may be reproduced, stored in
a retrieval system, or transmitted in any form or by any means, electronic,
mechanical, photocopying, recording or otherwise without the prior permis-
sion of the copyright owners.

First published by the authors themselves.
2009

This book is dedicated to our wonderful patients from whom we have learned so much, to the members of the International Academy of Oral Medicine and Toxicology (IAOMT) with special mention to Dr Rich Fischer DDS MIAOMT, Dr David Kennedy DDS MIAOMT and the late Dr Michael Ziff DDS, former Director of the IAOMT. We are grateful for their support and expert knowledge over the years.

Disclaimer

Toxic Dentistry Exposed is for informational purposes only. The theories and practices explained are based on the personal opinions of the authors. The contents of the book are based on scientific literature and the experience of the authors. The contents of the book do not reflect mainstream opinion of either medicine or dentistry; at least, not yet. Nothing in this book is intended to diagnose or treat any disease or condition. It is neither medical nor dental advice, nor should it be construed as such. Always seek the opinion of the relevant qualified health professional before making any changes to your diet, prescription drug use, lifestyle, exercise activities or prior to undergoing any dental procedure.

THE AUTHORS

Dr Graeme Munro-Hall BDS FIAOMT

Graduated in 1971 at University of St. Andrews. Between 1977 and 1981 he successfully completed the full programme at the LD Pankey Institute for Advanced Dental Education in Miami, USA . In 1984 he became a mercury-free dentist. He became a member of the IAOMT in 1989 and was awarded a fellowship for pioneering work in safe dental treatment in 1993.

Dr Lilian Munro-Hall BDS

Born in Denmark. She graduated in 1988 from Lund University in Sweden. She has worked in various countries around the world and speaks five languages.

Together they have developed the V-Tox therapy for safe dental treatment after extensive investigations into pH, diet, dental toxins and infections. In 1999 they started the first orthomolecular dental clinic in the UK offering the safest dental treatment possible. They were among the first to aquire a Cavitat scanner in Europe. The Cavitat has shown that dental infections are a far more serious problem than first thought. Dental toxins from metals and infections can be extremely damaging to health.

CONTENTS

8 YOU ARE UNDER ATTACK

9 WHAT DO I DO NOW?

LIST OF CASE STUDIES

INDEX

FOREWORD I

If you are reading this, you are probably concerned about your own health, or the health of someone you care about. You may have investigated or even tried many different approaches, both 'orthodox' or 'alternative', in your endeavour to overcome the ill-health you have been struggling with. Perhaps you have begun the journey back to health, and are exploring resources which can support this, or perhaps you are feeling desperate and looking for how to start on this path. You are not alone.

Our human species is becoming burdened with the consequences of an increasing load of 'legal' environmental toxins, which the immune system struggles to cope with. In order to try and deal with the burgeoning array of modern chronic diseases (MCDs) which result from this, yet more poisons are administered by people who have signed the Hippocratic Oath. What is going on?

ORTHODOX MEDICINE

The word 'healing' comes from the Old English word *hælan*, which in turn has roots in more ancient languages, meaning 'to make whole, sound and well'. Suppressing or controlling symptoms with drugs generates ill-health which eventually becomes 'normalised'. Mainstream medical practice, embedded as it is in the culture within which it operates, cannot but be influenced by prevailing beliefs, attitudes and values. And it in turn exerts its own influence. Take a look at the world as it is today, and realise that what you see is not the result of a healing attitude which respects the life of the human, animal, plant and mineral kingdoms which inhabit this earth. Sadly, it is to the contrary.

'Quacks'

Note that the word 'quack' is short for quacksalver, from the Dutch kwaksalver, meaning 'hawker of salve', referring to one who 'quacked' in the market-place about his 'medical' wares, some of which were harmless but ineffective, others of which could be poisonous, like arsenic or mercury. Although the word 'salve' also refers to 'ointment', the obvious similarity with the word quicksilver cannot be ignored. Note that quackery also has an ancient association with magic, alchemy and stage spectacles, including those of travelling preachers – people who create illusion. For those who today peddle dental mercury and manage to beguile the public into false reassurance about its harmlessness have indeed an ancient and ignoble pedigree associated with quackery.

THINK 'OUTSIDE THE BOX'

The principles of mainstream healing and health have been hijacked by the persuasive marketing techniques of the pharmaceutical industry. Doctors and dentists who have a true healing vocation are being routinely betrayed by the commercial interests now firmly vested in their own 'profession', which they in turn collude with, knowingly or otherwise. Today, however, there is no excuse. There is an enormous amount of information in the public domain which was previously hidden from medical professionals and patients alike. However, it takes a great deal of courage for any medical professional to think 'outside the box', start 'joining up the dots', seeing the obvious and acting accordingly. At best, he or she risks misunderstanding or ridicule; at worst, approbation, ostracization, or even outright persecution. This is exactly the kind of courage that has been portrayed by Drs Graeme and Lilian Munro-Hall, who have dedicated their entire professional lives to discovering and practising the kind of truth that really does result in healing and curing, even in cases which have confounded 'medical science'.

THE FUTURE OF MAINSTREAM MEDICINE

Today, following the truth of the natural, obvious, healing ways is no longer a matter of choice, but of survival – and it requires of us a radical 'paradigm shift'. The good news is that this is possible, as illustrated by the many moving stories in this book. There are indeed healing procedures available which will support, rather than destroy, your health. The medicine of the future will be a combination of scientific technique, as needed, and a sound naturopathic understanding of the need for radical detoxification, the curing of infection and the intelligent support of the body's capacity to heal itself.

THE FUTURE IS NOW

The Munro-Halls are among a growing number of pioneers on this path, which represents a truly 'holistic' way of healing. We are talking about nothing less than a revolution as we wake up from the collective 'trance' induced by the false claims of medical orthodoxy, backed up by 'research' often funded by those who stand to profit from their 'conclusions'.

If you have read this far, the chances are that this material touches a chord within you. As you read further, prepare to feel shocked and also deeply relieved as you hear someone finally telling the truth and talking sense, in particular about dentistry-related health issues, but also offering wisdom and practical advice which will support your healing.

Melanie Reinhart, author of *Chiron and the Healing Journey*

FOREWORD II

Some 20 years ago I was introduced to the 'amalgam wars' shortly after I published some papers showing that exposing age-matched, normal human brain tissue to mercury caused the same abnormal biochemistry as also observed in the Alzheimer's diseased brain. Colleagues and I repeated this experiment by having rats breathe mercury vapor with the same abnormal biochemistry appearing.

The reaction to our data, published in respected scientific journals was remarkable. I was castigated and accused of being a radical, junk scientist even though my NIH funding and publication records were good. The attacks came primarily from the dental industry and were symptomatic of a group trying to protect an important income stream or to escape serious lawsuits.

Since that time I have worked to resolve the problem of amalgam filling toxicity and was noted for making the statement: 'I feel I have been in an eight-year argument with the town drunk.' It is now 20 years and no progress has been made with our federal health agencies as the FDA (Food and Drug Administration of America) recently concluded that amalgam fillings were safe to be placed in all humans, even those on kidney dialysis, pregnant, ill from infections, etc.

This is why this book is needed and timely. We are in an age where our government health agencies work to protect the income of the industries and trade unions in the dental and medical fields and the safety of the patients takes a back seat if it is considered at all. This book details the dangers of mercury exposure from dental amalgams, some of the politics involved and is on target to help the patients who are seeking an improvement in their health, which has been negatively affected by years of breathing toxic mercury vapor from their amalgam fillings.

Prof Boyd Haley, Emeritus Professor of Chemistry of the University of Kentucky

INTRODUCTION

ABOUT THE AUTHORS
Graeme Munro-Hall

I started life as a conventional drill, fill and bill dentist. This meant working with amalgam and gold and doing exactly as I was taught in dental school. It was patch and repair dentistry with little intrinsic satisfaction to it.

Heart trouble

In my late twenties, I was at an ADA (American Dental Association) conference in the USA where I was offered a cardiac check up. I stood in line for the Electrocardiography (ECG), blood pressure (BP), and weight and height measurements to be taken; and then off to see the nurse for evaluation. Ten minutes after my measurements had been taken, I was in front of the nurse who, glancing at the data, told me to see the cardiac specialist in the neighbouring booth NOW. I was the only one selected for this out of a long line of far more elderly dentists than myself. As I felt perfectly okay, I wondered why I had been selected, but knew it was not for my sparkling personality or good looks!

The cardiologist examined the ECG, listened to the heart, and told me that the horizontal axis of my heart had moved and that with a BP of 185 over 135, I must have a blood test for triglycerides. When the blood test came back, it showed massively high levels of 'bad' cholesterol, all predisposing factors for a large, probably fatal, heart attack. Furthermore, all these indications were a sign of stress on the heart and that I needed to do something about it urgently, although he could not suggest exactly what should or could be done.

The medical solution

Back in the UK, I took these results to another cardiologist – a kind elderly man. All he could say was that I was at risk of a heart attack earlier rather than later. He could only offer the advice of reducing

V

stress and taking BP reducing tablets. I did not feel that I was under excessive stress, neither did I want to rely on tablets to suppress one part of the symptoms for the rest of the time left to me, which he estimated at between 5 and 10 years. Also, the side-effects of the available medication would reduce the quality of these 5 to 10 years remaining, not extend my life span. It would be better to do nothing and enjoy what I had left. I had seen what had happened to others on such a regime and I was not convinced it was actually helpful except to the financial interests of the drug company. This was neither encouraging nor very helpful, so essentially I was on my own.

My own solution

My problems were entirely due to mercury from dental amalgam. As well as having amalgam and gold fillings, I had been using amalgam on a daily basis without any protection since I was a student at dental school. I had my amalgam and other dental metals removed using a form of the metal removal protocol which we use now on our patients. Although at the time, I put myself in the position of an experimental guinea pig, I not only survived the removal but also felt better. I knew then that we were onto something significant.

The fact that I am here today over 60 years of age with a BP of 125 over 80, a blood chemistry the envy of a 30-year-old, no thickening of the arteries, the heart back in its place and a low cholesterol level, is wholly as a result of all our own efforts and research.

Lilian Munro-Hall
THROMBOSIS AND ALLERGIES

Lilian's example was different. In her early 40s, she awoke one day with a thrombosis in the arm. She became suddenly allergic to a host of substances. Blood tests revealed skyrocketing liver enzyme values, which signified the breakdown of liver cells. This came as a shock to someone who drank little alcohol, never smoked, and exercised regularly.

The medical solution

Symptom suppression was the only suggestion that conventional doctors could offer. The alternative route of auto-vaccines for the allergies just would have made matters worse, as is usually the case.

Lilian's solution

Tests showed Lilian's problem to be a reaction to palladium in a crown which was fixed to a root-filled tooth, and not mercury based at all. So her problem was due to a dental metal: palladium; and an infected root-filled tooth, both done 6 years earlier.

Removal of this tooth in the correct manner solved Lilian's problems quickly and permanently which was something no medical intervention whether conventional or alternative could have done.

Both of our life threatening medical conditions were due entirely to the effects of conventional dentistry and both were reversed by applying sensible scientific holistic dental protocols. 'It is not rocket science, just housewives' commonsense', to quote Lilian.

ABOUT THE BOOK

The contents of this book may seem controversial to some. However, all that is stated here is based on science published in accredited journals and the results of our own experience in applying this knowledge in everyday practice on large numbers of sick patients. All the case histories in this book are from our own files as are all the clinical photographs. We are not armchair warriors, but practising dentists endeavouring to do our best for our patients and to let other dentists have access to our knowledge and experience. We know what works and on what type of patient it is effective.

Chapters

This book is divided into sections. At the end of each section, there will be a summary of the contents so that readers can easily recap what they have read and also refer to the summary when reading other sections.

Caution: Before having any work done, consult the appropriate health care professional. Do not rush into treatment. Successful treatment is like a ballroom dance: to be effective it has to be performed in sequence, each step following the other. Failure to follow the sequence can make a bad situation a lot worse.

CHAPTER 1

The 'what, how and why': the causes of modern chronic diseases, how it all started, and why.

CHAPTER 2

The solution to the problems illustrated in Chapter 1, outlining diagnosis and practical treatments that can be applied.

CHAPTER 3

A series of case studies, actual patient treatments we have done, showing what treatment was done, why, how it succeeded and over what time frame. All the case studies are chosen from patients we have treated. This includes the photographs, illustrations and laboratory results to show the variety of conditions that can be helped in this way.

CHAPTER 4

This 'panic chapter' is for patients who have been recently given a diagnosis of a serious condition and are panicking over what to do. The panic chapter is for those in a hurry and can be read first but not to the exclusion of the first three parts.

CHAPTER 5

A practical application of Chapter 2, The Solution: shows actual case histories of how to treat neurological conditions, allergies, multiple chemical sensitivities, ME and chronic fatigue, irritable bowel syndrome, psoriasis, eczema, dermatitis, hair-thinning, anxiety, depression, obsessive compulsive disorder (OCD), panic attacks, irritability, short-term memory loss, brain fog, lack of concentration and loss of confidence, heart and cardio vascular disorders, arthritis, rheumatoid arthritis, ankylosing spondylitis, multiple sclerosis, Sjögren's syndrome, Hashimoto's thyroiditis, chronic iritis, glaucoma, and the 'unlabelled' patient.

CHAPTER 6

This chapter discusses cancer and infertility, both of which are dramatically increasing in modern society. For cancer, the emphasis is on prevention rather than cure. Infertility can affect both males and females and needs to be regarded as a modern chronic disorder rather than a disease entity.

CHAPTER 7

The how and why the problems with toxicity and MCDs were allowed to happen. It shows ways of protecting yourself and your family.

CHAPTER 8

As a dentist, medical doctor or as a patient, the question is, 'What do I do now?' This chapter addresses this question.

WHO THIS BOOK IS FOR

The book is aimed at the open-minded information seeking patient rather than the dentist. As such, it is written in fairly non-technical terms for ease of understanding. Scientific references can be found at www.toxicdentistryexposed.com.

Note: The website associated with this book will give more up-to-date and detailed information than is possible with the limited space available here.

CAN CONVENTIONAL PRACTITIONERS HELP YOU?

It does require experience to know what tests to organise, how to read the results and organise the sequence of events required to bring the patient back to health.

Whether this co-ordinator is a medical doctor or a dentist or another knowledgeable health professional, does not really matter. What does matter, is the knowledge, skill, experience and attitude of those doing the work. It is not something your average dentist or doctor can do, or is even interested in doing; it is work far beyond their professional comfort zone. As proponents of allopathic or conventional medicine, dentistry will not willingly admit they are wrong.

> 'Most men can seldom accept even the simplest and most obvious truth if it would oblige them to admit the falsity of conclusions which they have delighted in explaining to colleagues, have proudly taught to others, and have woven thread by thread into the fabric of their lives.'
>
> Tolstoy

WE CAN HELP

Life is supposed to be joyful with energy and vitality. If your life is not like this, the information in this book may help you regain it. There is no magic bullet; only common sense, effort and dedication will work. No-one can give the solution to you. Your mind is like a parachute: you obtain the best results when it is open.

> **Note:** It does not matter what label has been placed on a patient in most cases. Our experience is that 80% of patients will gain significant improvement by following the advice in this book. The remaining 20% may require other tricks we have learnt over the years to achieve improvement in their health. Some patients are, of course, beyond help.

Drs Graeme and Lilian Munro-Hall

X

MODERN CHRONIC DISEASE: THE 'WHAT, HOW AND WHY'

WHAT ARE MODERN CHRONIC DISEASES?

Modern chronic diseases (MCDs) are an epidemic sweeping across both first and third world countries. By MCDs, we mean both the dramatic increase in long established conditions, such as cancer and depression, as well as the new kids on the block, such as Alzheimer's. Asthma, chronic fatigue syndrome, syndrome x, multiple chemical sensitivity, allergies, ankylosing spondylitis, arthritis, dermatitis, psoriasis, plus many more are all on the increase and are examples of MCDs.

Patient conditions or labels

Patients come with all sorts of labels or diagnoses put on them. Here is a sample; the list is not exhaustive:

NEUROLOGICAL	IMMUNE DISORDERS
Peripheral neuropathy	Sjorgren's disease
Multiple sclerosis	Hashimoto's thyroiditis
Autism	Arthritis
Alzheimer's	Ankylosing spondylitis
Parkinson's	Chronic iritis
Motor neurone disease	Irritable bowel
	Crohn's disease

1

MENTAL CONDITIONS	ALLERGIC CONDITIONS
Anxiety	Chronic fatigue (CFS)
Depression	Multiple chemical sensitivity
Confusion	(MCS)
Excessive shyness	Asthma
Memory loss	Dermatitis
Aggression	Allergies
Obsessive compulsive behaviour	Food sensitivities
	Fibromyalgia
Phobias	Rashes
CANCER	CHRONIC INFLAMMATION
All types	(the forerunner for all MCDs)
	Varicose veins
	Bleeding gums
	Haemorrhoids
	Hernia
	Connective tissue disorders
HEART AND CIRCULATION	REPRODUCTIVE DIFFICULTIES
Abnormal cholesterol levels	Infertility male and female
Heart attacks	Endometriosis
Strokes	Premenstrual tension
	Irregular and painful periods

This list by no means all-inclusive, we can add light and electrical sensitivity, balance difficulties, tinnitus, hearing loss, altered vision, sense of smell, diabetes etc.; almost ad infinitum.

PATIENTS WITH NO LABELS OR 'IT'S ALL IN YOUR HEAD'

Many patients have no labels on their symptoms. Often the patient has many symptoms which defy diagnosis. These are the most unfortunate patients. If they had a broken leg, the plaster splint would be visible to all. However, because the symptoms are not immediately visible and they have no diagnosis or label, they are not taken seriously enough. Unfortunately it can be, and often is, worse than that. These patients are told, 'It is all in your head' and they should, 'Buck up and pull themselves together'. The horrible reality is that these patients feel alone and abandoned often wondering whether it really is in their heads when the reality is that they are poisoned through no fault of their own.

CASE STUDY 1

The symptoms and causes

This family had run out of options. Mother and father in their fifties: the mother with chronic pain in the gut, the father retired early due to heart disease. Both parents had amalgam fillings and root-filled teeth. The oldest child was in her mid-twenties and housebound with chronic fatigue. She had seven amalgam fillings and four infected wisdom teeth. The youngest child was in his twenties and had given up university due to chronic fatigue that started after having two wisdom teeth removed 18 months earlier which had turned into cavitation infections. He also had seven amalgam fillings.

The treatment

All of them went through the same treatment process of an individualised supplementation programme based on their pH levels. After which, they had the amalgams correctly removed at the same time as high dose Vitamin C infusions were administered. The infected teeth were removed and the cavitation infections cleaned. The treatment was correctly carried out under the V-Tox protocol which is described later in the book (see page 95).

The recovery
    The end result was that both the children rebounded
into health, going to university and graduating, and improved health and function for the parents. The children
could lead normal lives, have jobs, get married and they
did. Their symptoms were but a distant memory. Without
the correct treatment outlined in this book, it is doubtful
whether any of this could have happened.

It is for families like this that book has been written. Health can
be restored in most cases even when conventional and alternative
medicine has given up on you. Just a case of 'housewives common
sense' – If you are poisoned, you are going to get sick.

THE CONVENTIONAL SOLUTION

Conventional medicine has nothing to offer, no matter how sympathetic the doctor is. The patient is sent to multiple specialists for
lots of expensive and exhausting tests. All the tests come back as
'normal' and the quest for help goes on until the patient runs out of
patience, money or specialists to go to. The same scenario can be
repeated with the patient seeing a host of alternative practitioners as
well. As one patient succinctly said, 'I have spent $10,000 on tests
for doctors to tell me I am sick, but I already knew that'. Until the
root cause of the problem is sensibly addressed, no treatment will
offer long-term success.

Conventional treatment, such as it exists today, is almost solely
concerned with trying to reduce the effect of symptoms. These usually
consist of drugs to reduce the immune system response, steroid drugs
like prednisolone, cortisone etc. These drugs, when used for multiple sclerosis for example, can be very useful but they are concerned
purely with symptom relief, making life easier in the short-term for
the patient. They should not be taken long-term due to the side-effects
of thinning skin, moon face and an increased risk of cancer. They are,

4

after all, immune system suppressors and suppressing your immune defences is bound to give you trouble eventually.

Other drugs are to prevent muscle twitching or pain in muscles. Even giving L-Dopa to Parkinson's patients works only for a limited time, usually very effective in the beginning, but after a while only the negative aspects of the drug remain and all positive responses have gone for ever. None of the treatments or drugs, which conventional medicine utilises, address the root cause of modern chronic disease and so no long-lasting relief is available to the patient.

HOW TO 'CURE' MCDS

Let us be perfectly clear at the outset that there is *no cure* for any of these diseases. There is no pill or potion that can take away the cause. Symptomatic relief may be possible with pills and potions, but the underlying cause is seldom touched by modern drugs. Modern conventional medicine and dentistry are more likely to be part of the problem than part of the solution. Medicine and dentistry are capable of adding to the overall toxic load on a patient rather than reducing it. The toxic materials and methods employed by modern dentistry are explained in Chapter 3 (see page 35). Symptom reduction rather than disease elimination is the order of the day.

> 'It is the job of the doctor to amuse the patient whilst he cures himself.'
>
> Voltaire

This is as true today as when Voltaire first said it, but today's doctor usually adds to the toxic load of the patient with drugs which makes it more difficult for the patient to cure himself.

However, identifying and removing the toxic insults from the body in a controlled manner will *allow the body to heal itself.* Sometimes of course, the damage done to the body by the toxins is so great that it is beyond the capacity of the body to repair itself. In these cases, after treatment, the condition either slows down, which is usual, or continues as before. There is no way of measuring where this point of no return is for any individual. That being the case, it is always worthwhile removing the toxins to at least give the patient a chance of recovery. We have witnessed even the most seemingly hopeless cases recover when given the chance. The only solution is a true holistic approach as described in detail in Chapter 4 (see page 94).

This simple concept is contrary to medical belief which has spent years categorising and labelling symptoms.

> 'It is important to remember that the name put on any disease or the symptoms expressed will vary according to the genetic make up of the patient, the nature of the toxins and the length of time the patient is exposed to the toxins.'
>
> Drs G and L Munro-Hall

It does not matter what label has been placed on a patient in most cases. Our experience is that 80% of patients will gain significant improvement by removing the toxins in the correct manner and supporting the body's healing mechanisms alone. The remaining 20% may require other tricks we have learnt over the years to improve their condition.

> 'No healing can occur until the proper nutrition is in place, the toxins removed and the infections dealt with. Unless this is done, correctly, safely and in the right order, all treatment is only suppressing symptoms.'
>
> Drs G and L Munro-Hall

If the correct environment is created in the body by good nutrition and removal of the toxins and infections, the body can heal itself without further intervention.

> 'No drug or doctor can cure any condition.'
>
> Drs G and L Munro-Hall

Read that again, it is vital to grasp this point. The best any of us can do, no matter what approach to illness and treatment we use, is to create the conditions to allow healing to take place, **provided** the body still has the capacity to heal. Whether a body still has the capacity to heal or has gone past the point of no return is impossible to measure. The capacity of any patient to heal cannot be measured; we have seen enough amazing recoveries from seemingly hopeless situations to know that there is always hope.

CASE STUDY 2

A young woman came to us with an unlabelled but progressive neurological condition. After one year of having this condition, she was on a respirator full time and only able to move one finger. Within three months of her toxin removal, done properly, she was sitting up in bed chatting to us, which was something even we believed would have been impossible when we started the treatment.

The story unfortunately does not have a happy ending. About a year later, after slow but steady progress, she went to a British hospital for a check up; caught an infection in the hospital and died there within 48 hours.

THE CAUSES OF MCDS
1. Toxins

In brief, toxic insults to the body from chemical or viral/bacterial/fungal sources, usually in combination, are behind the explosion of MCDs. The symptom or manifestation of these toxins on a particular patient will depend on the nature of the toxin and the individual genotype. In other words, specific toxins acting on an individual over time will cause a symptom due to the genetic make up or weakness of that individual.

One person under the same toxic influence may have multiple sclerosis symptoms, whereas another individual with different genes

7

may have a psychosis. The cause is the same in both cases, but the symptoms and the labels are different.

> **Note:** MCDs are caused by the build up of toxins which, in time, overwhelm the body's detoxification and defence system. The quantity and type of toxin acting on the specific genotype of the patient will dictate what symptoms are shown. The same toxin in different patients can show entirely different symptoms.

Exposure on a daily basis to an ever increasing load of toxins eventually overwhelms the capacity of the body to deal with them. This exposure is from food, water, medicines, the general environment, and above all dentistry. These toxins cause, amongst other things, a low oxygen utilisation. Heavy metals, such as mercury and cadmium used in dentistry, can adversely affect cellular function in a variety of ways, as can transitional metals such as titanium. Such metals are toxins in their own right. Toxins alone, acting on a weakened body which has an incorrect pH, can cause a breakdown of the normal bodily functions and disease processes will start. In absolute terms, the quantity of toxins released by toxic dentistry may be small, but the damaging effects of the toxins on the body can be enormous.

> 'Symptoms produced are out of proportion to the amount of toxin released and can be anywhere or in any system of the body'.
>
> Dr Weston Price

THE EFFECT OF YEARS OF POISONING

All modern chronic diseases are not handed down from on high by chance to unfortunate individuals or from one day to the next. They arise from the chronic poisoning of the patient over the years. The symptoms displayed by the patient are a result of the types, the concentration and the duration of exposure to toxins. The mixture of the toxins and the genetic weaknesses of the patient determine what symptoms arise. The same exposure of toxins that give one patient

8

Parkinson's, may give another MCD, and no overt symptoms to yet another. The labels patients have are interesting only for the type of symptoms that will be displayed and the rate of progression of the illness.

A sudden event can cause a catastrophic onset of symptoms. Minor surgery, a metal filling or exposure to a toxin can seem to act as a trigger, but it is a mistake to attribute the event to the immediate release of the toxin. What has happened is that over the preceding years, the reserve of the body to cope with toxins has been reduced until the day comes that there is no reserve capacity left to protect the body. When this happens, even the smallest event can have the most dramatic consequences. Most often the symptoms were coming on gradually, but occasionally a sudden event caused the start of the symptoms.

Imagine you are walking along a cliff top by the seaside. You admire the view, breathe in the air, everything is fine. Yet all the time you are walking, you are being pushed just the smallest bit towards the edge. You seldom notice the pushes and even if you do, you can shrug it off, call it getting older, and get on with the walk. Eventually, after enough pushes, you are walking right on the very edge of the cliff. You still feel fine, everything is as it was and should be. Then, with you teetering on the edge of the cliff, another tiny push comes along. This time you go over the cliff and down you fall.

This catastrophic consequence was due to the sum of all the pushes not just the last one. Removing the last push, if that were possible, will not bring you back to the cliff top, you are lying, a mangled wreck, at the bottom of the cliff. You want to get back to the top of the cliff but when the rescue services arrive, they shake their heads, offer you a pain killer and tell you that, sooner or later depending on your injuries, you are going to die. Sometimes of course, the fall off the cliff is a fatal stroke or heart attack and sudden death is the result. The heart attack did not arise from the last pack of cigarettes smoked but was due to the cumulative effect of all the packs of cigarettes smoked over the last 20 years in combination with an antioxidant deficient diet.

What you have to do is find someone to throw you a rope and make you strong enough to climb the rope back up the cliff top. When you are finally up on top of the cliff, and a superhuman effort it is too, you must take care to walk well away from the edge. You must take great efforts to avoid all pushes towards the cliff edge or the same thing will happen again, and if it does, you are unlikely to have the strength to climb up the rope once more. This book is your starting point to finding the rope you need to climb up the cliff into health.

THE KINDLING RESPONSE

It is pertinent to remember here that the body has a memory and this is called a 'kindling response'. What this means is that any stresses on the body in the future, from whatever cause, will create the same symptoms that you originally suffered because the body 'remembers' that this is how it responded to past stresses.

Cancer treatment is a good illustration of this point. How many times have you heard of the cancer patient being operated on, burnt with radiation and poisoned with chemotherapy, the cancer 'success-fully' treated, only for it to come roaring back a few years later on? Unless the cause of the original cancer was dealt with, of course it is going to come back; and it is exactly the same with other chronic illnesses or MCDs.

In order to return to health, to walk on top of the cliff, you have to deal with the all the root causes of your condition. This takes time and effort. It takes time to look into your past medical/dental history, environmental and mental issues, and identify what needs to be addressed.

It takes great effort to find the right health care provider that can guide you through the treatment maze to restored health. It takes even greater effort and steely determination to follow the correct treatment path often against the well meant advice of doctors and relatives.

The body has a large reserve capacity, this means that it can cope with a lot of damage before any symptoms show. However, when the symptoms do start, it means that a lot of damage has already occurred. Reversing this damage is usually a long process. No-one gets ill overnight and no-one recovers overnight either. Recovery time is proportional to the toxicity and length of time of exposure to the toxins, as well as the genetic make up and mental attitude of the patient. The principles of all this were first explained by Hans Selye in his book *The Stress of Life*. He justly received a Nobel Prize for this work.

POISONING VERSUS SENSITIVITY AND ALLERGY

Toxins can cause two problems for the body: poisoning, and sensitivity or allergic responses. They can appear separately or together. This causes endless confusion to the healing professions.

> **Remember the mantra:** Remove all the toxins and create the conditions for the body to heal itself.

- **Poisoning** is dose dependant. This means the more you are exposed to the poison, the worse the effect of the poison has on you. Poisons slow and shut down the body's functioning systems. They interfere with feedback mechanisms, corrupt messenger molecules, stop oxygen utilisation and a host of other things according to their properties.
- **Allergic** or sensitivity responses are not dose dependant. The toxin, even in minute amounts, triggers the immune system into a reaction. This can be seen from a skin rash to irritable bowel syndrome or chronic fatigue syndrome, or a host of other reactions.

Most patients will have both poisoning and sensitivity responses to various toxins.

2. Poor nutrition

Insufficient minerals and vitamins, too few good fats, too many bad fats and processed foods give the body the wrong pH environment to work in. This reduces the effectiveness of the body systems to deal with infections and toxins. A weakened immune system is a good example. Most of the patients are suffering from nutritional deficits of one sort or another that reduces their healing capacity and makes a bad situation a lot worse.

If you have an infection you will be using a higher amount of vitamins and minerals than you would do in normal circumstances. If the nutrients are not available in the body, healing is delayed. Similarly if you are nutritionally bankrupt, and most people are, your initial defence against infection is reduced making it easier for you to get an infection, be it viral, bacteria or fungal which can gain a foot-hold somewhere in the body. The direct and indirect action of these infections, releasing toxins, can be enough to cause a catastrophic breakdown of health.

3. Stress

Stress, or rather 'distress', be it structural, mental, or from infec-tions weakens the immune system of the body, which can allow disease to get a foothold. Toxins, poor nutrition, and distress are interconnected with each other. One lowers the resistance to the others.

For instance, it is well known that a depressed and anxious patient, or one with a negative mental attitude, has less resistance to illness than a patient with a happy positive attitude. The mental state of the patient reduces their resistance to infection.

Brilliantly described by Candice Pert in her book *Molecules of Emotion*, the mental state of a patient has a direct effect on the physical working of the body. A depressed patient has a depressed metabolism and a depressed immune system. All these factors lower the resistance to infection, as well as chemical and metal toxins. One of the toxic effects of mercury released from dental amalgam is depression so a downwards vicious cycle of ill health is easily set in motion.

STRESS FROM INFECTIONS

What about infectious diseases such as Lyme's which manifest themselves as chronic fatigue and allergies etc.? Similarly, what about malaria or measles for that matter?

There are two sides to infectious conditions: the immune defences of the patient, and the infectious organism. Most of these infections are opportunistic, they can only attack and gain a foothold if the immune defences of the patient are not up to par. The immune defences can be weakened by toxins. So the infection is an indication of a deeper problem in the patient: toxic overload, rather than a random event.

12

Certainly the specific organism must be targeted, but unless the underlying problem is solved, obviously it is only a matter of time before another bad health event occurs. What we maintain is that for the majority of patients, removing the toxins in a prescribed manner is, by itself, enough to solve most health and infective situations. The body can mobilise its defences and do what it needs to do to recover optimum health. A body loaded with toxins is fighting a battle with one hand tied behind its back. So the organism behind the label of the patient's disease is only a minor factor in treating the patient. The patient's body knows better how to recover optimum health than we ever can, so creating the conditions that allow the patient to recover optimum health is the first thing to do. Remove the toxins in the prescribed manner and make sure the nutritional status of the patient is excellent.

Targeting the organism or treating the symptom is part of any treatment. This does not always mean short- or long-term antibiotics. Indeed, for Lyme's this can be counterproductive. Malaria, and other insect transmitted diseases, can be considered broadly similar to Lyme's. Measles is entirely a different matter. Childhood illnesses play an important role in developing a mature functioning immune system in the adult. The suppression of such childhood illnesses by vaccines is, in the authors view, detrimental to long-term health. It would appear that the measles virus has mutated in the vaccine to be far more virulent that the 'normal' measles virus. This, and the weaker nature of modern children compared to their parents due to toxic load, would explain the greater severity of the disease now.

CASE STUDY 3

The symptoms

A female patient in her early 50s with three children and a political and working career, had found it more and more difficult to cope as time went on. Symptoms started with loss of smell at age eight after her first amalgam fillings. For the last 15 years, she had chronic fatigue and

13

was unable to go on holiday, often even unable to get out of bed. She found herself housebound most of the time. Multiple allergies, which were increasing in severity, had been present for many years; she had frequent urinary and respiratory infections. No conventional or alternative regime had helped at all during this time.

She was a lifelong non-smoker, little alcohol consumption (typically these patients have very low alcohol tolerance), with an organic sensible diet (no fast or convenience foods), some supplementation, and lots of good quality water consumed. Innumerable tests had been performed at great expense over the years, but the reason for her condition remained a mystery to modern medicine. Her only offers of treatment from her medical advisors were antibiotics, tranquilisers, anti-depressants and steroids; all of which she sensibly declined.

The causes

Examination showed two amalgam fillings, one gold inlay, three metal (nickel-based stainless steel) pins under the amalgam fillings, two composite fillings, five metal ceramic crowns (made from non-precious metal alloys), and three root-treated teeth. She also had **structural** stress: The 'bite' was near collapse; it was over-closed and both jaw joints were pushed back into the skull. There was no anterior freedom and she had group function on the back teeth. What this means is when she closed her mouth, the teeth came together and locked the jaw in one position. This caused the jaw muscles to go into spasm.

Stress in the form of **infection** was also present. Her pH was acidic, around 5.2 for saliva and 5.6 for urine with little fluctuation of the levels. Basal (body) temperature was 36.4°C, which was low. In most cases, where the urine pH is *higher* than the saliva pH, there is chronic infection somewhere in the body. These patients usually take longer to turn around, than patients with a more standard pH reading where the urine levels are lower than the saliva levels.

The treatment

The preparation phase consisted of supplementation given for the three weeks prior to treatment, along with dietary recommendations, in order to raise pH levels and start healing and sealing the gut. This was a complex dental restorative case, but in essence the root-filled teeth were extracted and all the metals replaced with non-metallic aesthetically pleasing material. The 'bite' was corrected, which involved finding the correct jaw relationships and teeth contacts. The missing teeth were replaced by fixed bridges. The cement used to place the restorations in position was the same material as the bridges.

At the same time as the dental work was being done (over two consecutive days) and for another three days afterwards, intravenous infusions of vitamin C with glutathione and minerals were given. The infusions consisted of 40g vitamin C, 400mg glutathione, with minerals (selenium etc.) diluted in lactated ringers. Supplementation was adjusted and continued for another 8 months. **This is the V-Tox treatment.**

The recovery

Within two weeks, there was a massive improvement of symptoms. Within four weeks, her sense of smell was back, the allergies were rapidly fading and the fatigue was not so severe. After five months, the patient reported that she had not felt so well since she was a child and had forgotten how good it was to feel this way with an almost total resolution of her symptoms. She was leading an active life again. This was in 2002 and the patient has remained at this increased level of health ever since. pH levels were raised and remained stable and the basal temperature went up by 0.4°C.

Heal and seal the gut, remove the metals, restore a functioning 'bite', remove the infections, and keep to a good diet was the key to restoring good health not experienced in years. She had a strong positive mental attitude and an open mind, all of which was vital as well to her healing response.

THEORY OF THE ORIGINS OF MODERN CHRONIC DISEASE

1. External toxins
Drugs, chemicals (such as hair dyes, pesticides, herbicides, fertilisers, household and personal care products), exhaust fumes etc.

+

2. Internal toxins
Mercury fillings, dental and medical metals, focal infections, trauma, incorrect jaw relationships

+

3. Digestive tract
Leaky gut, inflamed or infected gut, poor nutrition, poor absorption

↓

4. Liver and kidney
Defective detoxification mechanisms, build up of toxic load

+

5. Immune system
Wrong signals (auto-immune), cannot cope with toxic load

+

6. Chronic inflammation starts
pH disturbance (the acid/alkali balance), connective tissue effects

+

7. Genetic weakness of patient

↓

8. Modern chronic disease
MCD begins after a time, usually after many years.

Steps 1,2 and 3 lead to 4,5 and 6, which when added to 7, result in 8.

SUMMARY

- Modern chronic diseases (MCDs) are primarily caused by a build up of toxins from all sources in the body over time.
- These toxins are extremely potent and can cause severe symptoms out of all proportion to the quantity of toxin.
- Modern diets and poorly functioning digestive tracts reduce the ability to cope with toxins.
- Patients may have labels, such as MS or CFS or allergy, or no label at all. In all cases, it is the build up of toxins that is the root cause of the problem.
- Conventional medicine can only offer symptomatic relief and does not get to the root cause of the problem. The same can be said for many types of alternative medicine too.
- Identifying the nature of the toxic load, successfully removing the toxins, optimising nutrition, healing and sealing the gut, will allow the body to heal itself.

Simple, but not easy

2 MODERN CHRONIC DISEASE: THE TOXIN AND NUTRITION CONNECTION

WHAT ARE TOXINS?

The definition of a toxin according to the National Institute of Health (NIH) is 'any substance that can act as a poison'. This is a broad definition. The medical definition of a toxin is 'one of a number of poisons produced by certain plants, animals, and bacteria.' The term 'toxin' is frequently used to refer specifically to a particular protein produced by some higher plants, animals and pathogenic (disease-causing) bacteria. A toxin typically has a high molecular weight (as compared to a simple chemical poison), is antigenic (elicits an antibody response), and is highly poisonous to living creatures. The word 'toxin' was introduced to medicine in 1888 as a name for poisons made by infectious agents. In brief, we will use this definition.

> 'A toxin is anything that acts as a poison and can cause allergies.'
>
> Drs G and L Munro-Hall

Let us repeat the cause of MCDs. Modern chronic diseases of 'civilisation' are caused by three major factors:

1. Poor nutrition: Insufficient minerals and vitamins, too few good fats, too many bad fats and processed foods give the body the wrong pH environment to work in. This reduces the effectiveness of the body systems to deal with infections and toxins.

19

2. Exposure on a daily basis to an ever increasing load of toxins that eventually overwhelms the capacity of the body to deal with them.

3. Stress or rather distress, be it structural, chemical, mental, electrical or from infections. The above factors allow infection, be it viral, bacteria or fungal, to gain a foothold somewhere in the body. The direct and indirect action of these infections (e.g. releasing toxins) can be enough to cause a catastrophic breakdown of health. Toxins alone acting on a weakened body with an incorrect pH can cause a breakdown of normal bodily function and the disease process will start. The symptoms of this disease process will be out of proportion to the amount of toxin released and can be anywhere or in any system of the body.

Toxins can also be simple chemical poisons too, such as mercury, arsenic, fluoride, and even gold.

WHERE DO TOXINS COME FROM?

Man-made chemicals

The chemical toxins that make you sick have been mainly created by mankind in the last 150 years. They are the toxins of civilisation, created to fulfil perceived needs and for profit. Each year, approximately 10,000 new chemicals are released into the world with little effort made to see how they react with each other and their effect on us. In this category belong agrochemicals, medical and recreational drugs, cosmetics, petroleum-based products, plastics, household products and so on. You are born with at least 280 modern chemical toxins in your blood stream. In 2005, the non-profit Environmental Working Group published the results of a study on toxins found in newborn babies. After analyzing the blood of newborn babies from around the US, they discovered 287 chemicals and other toxins. One of the pesticides that turned up the most was a by-product of DDT – a pesticide banned in 1972.

From these 287 chemicals:
- 76 cause cancer in humans and animals;
- 94 are toxic to the brain and nervous system;
- 79 cause birth defects or abnormal development.

It is not just babies that have a high toxic load. Not too long ago, the Public Broadcasting Service (PBS) in the USA had a special programme on what toxins they found in the blood of one of their employees. They found 84 distinct chemicals, solvents and toxins that are known to be harmful to health. These chemical residues – termed the 'chemical body burden' – are present in every human being on this planet, regardless of where you live or what you do.

Dr Michael McCally of the Mt. Sinai School of Medicine in New York, who led the research team for PBS, made this comment, 'Current "normal" body burdens of dioxin and several other [chemicals] in humans are at or near the range at which toxic effects occur in laboratory animals.'

Note: What this means is that studies on animals show that the average person is carrying enough toxins in the body to cause serious health problems.

The diseases of civilisation are the direct and indirect consequence of these exposures in combination with inadequate nutrition and dehydration.

DENTISTRY

The metals and procedures used in dentistry also produce toxins. Mercury from amalgam, titanium from implants, palladium, gold, nickel, chrome, to mention just a few, can have toxic consequences on the unsuspecting patient. Dental procedures such as root fillings can also cause exposure to many toxic chemicals, formaldehyde is an example.

We must not forget the natural or biological toxins we can be exposed to: the infections and the toxins released by these infections. Focal infections are those that release toxins causing symptoms in parts of the body some distance away from the infection site. These can be from tooth extraction sites, cavitation infections, root fillings, dead teeth, and gum (periodontal) infections.

WATER

Fluoride

The worst toxin in water is *hydrofluorosilic* acid which is added to water in fluoridated areas in the belief that it stops tooth decay. This is the 'fluoride' that is put in the drinking water. Not only is this untested for safety, it is not even proven to reduce tooth decay. Fluoride can only reduce tooth decay by applying it around the teeth locally in order to kill the bacteria. It is like swallowing sunblock cream to prevent sunburn: an idiotic and damaging idea. No reputable science shows that drinking hydrofluorosilic acid 'enriched' water reduces tooth decay.

Hydrofluorosilic acid is an even bigger enzyme disrupter than fluoride itself (fluoride is also present as it results from the partial breakdown of hydrofluorosilic acid). Hydrofluorosilic acid increases the uptake of lead in the brain, whereas the old-fashioned sodium fluoride does not. Fluoride, which is an enzyme disrupter is stored in the bones. It causes premature aging and increases the risk of cancer by over 10%, that's the science; it also alters brain function which in certain racial groups leads to an increase in crime. This is how fluoride alters brain function. There is enough fluoride in a large tube of toothpaste to kill a seven-year-old child. Children have died swallowing fluoridated toothpaste.

Fluoride also increases the risk of cancer. Dr Dean Burke, chief scientist at the National Cancer Institute, stated under oath at a Congressional hearing, 'Nothing causes or makes cancer explode in the body faster than fluoride'. If you are a scientist in a laboratory and you want to turn a strain of cells cancerous, you can either turn down the oxygen to the bacteria or add fluoride. Dr Burke worked out that adding fluoride to the water would increase the cancer rate by at least 10%. No-one has challenged his figures. Even if fluoride added to the water was effective in reducing tooth decay, the increased risk of cancer is too high a price to pay. Fluoride is even a class 2 registered poison.

Chlorine and other chemicals

Tap water goes through processes to remove harmful bacteria, such as the addition of chlorine. Chlorine has shown itself to have toxic consequences in water, such as increasing the rate of colon cancer (according to the Centers of Disease Control and Prevention), but nothing is done to remove chemicals from the water; these include agricultural chemicals from the land and drugs. Where water is recycled, the drugs excreted in the urine remain as they are not filtered out. Drugs, such as female hormonal contraceptives, mind-altering Prozac (a drug containing fluoride), antibiotics, and so on, are regularly found in drinking water. These are drugs excreted in the urine of those who have been prescribed them.

Air

During human evolution, the body established defence mechanisms in the digestive tract and immune system to deal with toxin intake. However, there is no defence mechanism to protect us from airborne toxins. What we breathe in is immediately bio-available. To put it another way, what we breathe in, stays in. Mercury vapour from amalgam fillings is breathed into the lungs and within 20 seconds it is deposited in the brain. Synthetic fragrances are never broken down and are found in every breath of air we take anywhere in the planet. Volatile organic carbons (VOCs), from plug in dispensers and aerosols, used to 'freshen' homes are absorbed through the lungs. No wonder the longer time spent in the house, the higher the risk of cancer. 'Fragrances that change your world', a popular advert states. How right they are; unfortunately, the change is not for the better.

Add to this the toxins in cosmetics, such as lead in lipstick, bismuth (a heavy metal) in face powder; the fragrances in deodorants, hair dyes, insecticides, DDT in cotton clothing, fire retardants in furniture and clothing and you have a potent mix of toxins. Some of these chemicals have been tested for safety, but by no means all of them. *None of them have been tested for safety when combined with*

23

other chemicals, so no-one knows what the risks are or who is most at risk. Mercury reacts in the presence of lead, they are synergistic. This means that lead increases the toxicity of mercury by around four times and mercury increases the toxicity of lead by the same amount; a case of 1+1= 4. Lead used to be added to petrol, paints and used as the material in water pipes.

Exhaust fumes from cars contain particulates that accumulate in the lung and blood, but the use of palladium in the catalyst converter has put a fine mist of ultra fine palladium into the air. Since the introduction of this technology, the percentage of the population sensitive to palladium has more than doubled. As dentists become under more financial pressure, one way to reduce costs is to substitute gold for palladium. A patient with a palladium crown is exposed to palladium 24/7 which, in conjunction with palladium vapour from exhaust fumes, is adding fuel to the fire.

THE EFFECTS OF TOXINS

The effect of any toxic mixture on an individual will depend on the following:
1. Genetic predisposition
2. The number and type of toxins the individual is exposed to
3. The length of time of exposure to the toxin
4. The nutritional status of the individual

Evaluating the patient

Since accurately evaluating any of the above four on any individual patient is impossible, there is no way of correlating firmly any toxin or toxic mixture with any symptom or diagnosed condition a patient may have other than in very broad terms. For instance, exposure to mercury can cause serious neurological and mental problems but there is no way of proving that the exposure to mercury in an individual is the cause of his or her problem. All that can be said is that there is a *high degree of probability* for such an exposure to cause problems which is shown to be correct by our statistics. *There are no tests that can prove mercury or other metals are the cause of a problem in any*

24

one individual. The only indication that mercury is the cause of a problem would be to remove the mercury (or toxin) and see if the symptoms resolve. In order to establish that mercury was the cause of the symptoms, it would have to be reinserted into the patient and the same symptoms return. In the real world this is, of course, both unethical and impossible to do.

In treatment, therefore, the cherry picking of toxins for removal is neither the most sensible, nor the most effective approach. All toxins must be identified and removed as there is no way of knowing in an individual patient whether a particular toxin or a mixture of toxins is to blame for the symptoms displayed. Removing the straw from the camels back will not help mend the broken back. The entire load has to be removed and healing applied to the back to obtain a satisfactory result.

It also means dealing with the after-effects of the toxins. This will be repairing damaged tissues and getting enough tissue functional again to start the healing process latent in every body.

Remember: Remove the toxins and create the conditions for the body to heal itself.

There is a time when the damage to the organs and tissue function will be beyond the remaining repair capacity of the body. No-one knows where this point is in any one individual patient, but it is usually quite late on in the process. Even if the patient cannot be brought back to complete health, the progression of the disease can be stopped or dramatically reduced, which can be enough in itself for many patients.

Suffice it to say that in our experience, most MCDs and nearly all cancers have chronic oral infections somewhere in the background. This is dealt with later in the book.

Pasteur or Beauchamp?

Western medicine has followed the lead of Pasteur in the belief that the organism is the enemy to be controlled and attacked. Whilst this approach does have some merit, it is far too simplistic. What is more important is the condition of the host that allows the infection to gain a foothold in the first place. A strong host will easily defeat an organism, whereas a host weakened by toxic exposure may allow the organism to establish itself and further weaken the host. Since the organisms creating the toxins cannot be dealt with by drugs, the sensible approach is to strengthen the host as best we can as well as physically removing the infection. This is the Beauchamp rather than the Pasteur approach to infection.

Let us give an example: In a bad influenza epidemic, only around 5 to 10% of the population succumb to the infection and get flu. The other 90% must have been exposed to the virus but they did not suffer the symptoms of influenza. The question is, or ought to be, what is the difference between the two groups? Why was the immune system of the 90% more able to fend off the attack of the influenza virus than the 10%? This is never asked; the only interest is in the 10%. Why is this? Because the answer is, regretfully, that money can be made from the 10%, not the healthy 90% in our present medical-fiscal model.

THE RELATIONSHIP BETWEEN NUTRITION AND TOXINS

Exposure to toxins can reduce nutritional levels and reduced nutritional levels can make the effect of toxins a lot stronger. A downward spiral of health is started. For example, mercury particles from amalgam fillings can enter and get lodged in the gut. Once here, the mercury particles alter the gut bacteria because mercury is so toxic that only certain types of bacteria in the gut can survive. This altered gut flora allows the overgrowth of unwanted organisms causing a gut inflammation and a leaky gut. Foodstuffs that leak out of the gut react with the immune system, most of which sits behind the gut, so multiple allergies to food arise. All this increases the body's acidity which reduces its resistance to mercury overall. A vicious circle is created that over time will lead to a modern chronic disease. The answer to this situation is to remove the mercury from the teeth and body properly, replenish the gut flora and allow healing to take place.

Modern western diets

Most modern western diets are rich in sugar and poor on nutrients, such as minerals and vitamins. As a general rule, the population eats too much grain and protein and too little fresh fruit and vegetables. Even those on a good diet can be deficient due to the poor nutritional quality of modern food. This leads to low levels of essential minerals, such as selenium, magnesium, zinc etc., as well as low levels of vitamins, such as C, D and the Bs.

Modern agricultural practices have increased the level of chemicals in food, such as fertilisers, pesticides and herbicides and at the same time reduced the mineral and vitamin contents of the food considerably. The food industry adds more additives for flavour, colour and preservation, and processes the food reducing the nutritional value even further.

For instance, just look at the US Department of Agriculture's (USDA) nutritional values for fruits and vegetables today compared to 1975. Take a look at the loss of vitamins and minerals since 1975.

- Apples: vitamin A is down 41%.
- Sweet peppers: vitamin C is down 31%.
- Watercress: iron is down 88%.
- Broccoli: calcium and vitamin A are down 50%.
- Cauliflower: vitamin C is down 45%; vitamin B1 is down 48%; and vitamin B2 is down 47%.
- Collards greens: vitamin A is down 45%; potassium is down 60%; and magnesium is down 85%.

This degradation of basic foodstuffs has been going on since the 1930s. What this means is that it is nigh on impossible to maintain a correct level of nutrients for health without supplements unless you grow your own on good soil and without using chemicals.

Mono sodium glutamate (MSG) and aspartame are amongst the very worst flavour enhancers and sweeteners added to food and soft drinks from a health perspective. Anyone with the slightest concern for health should eliminate these chemicals from their diet immediately. These toxins are neuro-excitory toxins, usually at a low level in food, but it is the cumulative effect over time that is the concern of all this untested toxic mixture. These chemicals disrupt the brains signalling and feedback mechanisms. Having a complete food source that also acts as a cleanser and detoxifier is critical. It can mean the difference between health and happiness or a life cut short.

SELENIUM

Why this matters can be illustrated by the mercury-selenium connection. Mercury attaches itself to cells in the same place as selenium does. Given a choice between selenium and mercury, the body will choose selenium every time and mercury cannot attach. If there is not enough selenium available then mercury will attach itself to the cells instead and disrupt the proper functioning of the cell.

VITAMIN C

Low blood levels of vitamin C increases the thickening of deposits in the arteries, low blood levels of vitamin D increase the risk of cancer substantially and so on. There are many examples to choose from. These low levels of nutrients do not cause disease in themselves. For example, extremely low levels of vitamin C produce scurvy, whereas merely low levels of the vitamin produce the thickening of the arteries which may only become apparent years later in a heart attack.

SUGAR

Sugar is bad. Artificial sweeteners are worse. Sugar, whether it is white granulated or brown organic or called glucose, fructose, corn syrup, sucrose, malt, maple syrup and even alcohol, is still sugar. Sugar robs you of water, minerals and vitamins. It increases the risk of diabetes, high cholesterol, feeds cancer cells, cardiovascular disease, allergies, anxiety, osteoporosis to name just a few of the effects. Sugar is cheap and is added to lots of foods including fish and processed meat. Read labels and avoid sugar; it reduces your nutrient status and metabolic efficiency. It turns the body more acidic, i.e. it lowers the pH of the body.

A neighbour of ours, a food engineer by profession if you can imagine such a thing, once told me, 'No-one ever gets fired for making things sweeter'. This has led to increased sugar content in nearly all prepared foods. Even mustard and soused herring has sugar added and this has come about over the last few years. Some of the 'healthy' breakfast cereals have doubled their sugar content in the last 15 years. The absurd focus on fat-free or low-fat foods has led to a direct increase in the amount of sugar in food. No fat means no taste, so sugar is added to substitute sweetness for taste.

CANDIDA

Most conventional doctors believe that Candida, a fungal infection, is a harmless inhabitant of the human body. A very small minority of doctors and a lot of alternative practitioners believe that Candida is the root of all evil. *Both groups are mistaken.*

Candida is an opportunist but weak pathogen and a normal part of the gut flora. It can only exist and become a problem in acid pH environments. It lives in the gut and if the normal gut flora is disturbed, by antibiotics, mercury from amalgam fillings, or whatever, Candida can proliferate first in the intestine, then invade other tissues throughout the body. The answer to Candida infection is to create the correct pH levels throughout the body. This is done through a combination of diet, intelligent supplementation and toxin removal in the correct manner. Chronic fungal problems will need long-term probiotics (gut bacteria) therapy and sometimes electronic therapies. Our experience with Candida is that once the underlying issues have been attended to, i.e. toxins and pH, Candida is dealt with by the body's own defences and does not need specific targeting in the majority, but not all, of cases.

pH and health

pH is the level of acidity or alkalinity in the body. Blood pH is slightly alkaline at 7.34. If the blood drops below this level, it is called acidic even though, strictly speaking, a pH level of 7 is neutral. Cells communicate and function through electrical, chemical and hormonal processes. In order for these signalling mechanisms to work, the body's internal environment must be in a slightly alkaline state. If our body becomes too acidic, it adversely affects the functioning of

29

all its parts: heart cells, blood cells, brain cells, nerve cells, muscle cells, bone cells, even skin and hair cells.

THE FIRST SIGNS OF ACIDITY

When the body cannot properly dispose of excessive acids building up in the bloodstream, the body attempts to maintain proper pH balance by eliminating the excess acids through the kidneys, lungs and skin or by neutralizing the acids during the processes of digestion and cellular metabolism. However, when too much acid is produced, the body cannot keep pace. In an effort to protect vital organs, the body diverts the harmful acids to be stored in tissues, joints and bones. This might make the organs temporarily safe, but the diversion can cause joint and skeletal problems such as osteo- and rheumatoid arthritis and osteoporosis, as well as skin conditions such as dermatitis and eczema, and tissue problems such as chronic fatigue and fibromyalgia.

Osteoporosis

In an attempt to neutralize excess acids, the body draws on its store of alkalizing minerals. The bones contain calcium phosphate. The bones dissolve to access this phosphate which neutralizes the acid. The calcium is dumped where it can end up as tartar or calculus on the backs of teeth or in joints or cells where it is seen as free calcium.

This leads to osteoporosis. Osteoporosis is only found in modern societies. It is entirely due to increased acidity in the body from a variety of causes. It is never seen in societies with unprocessed foods and no access to modern medicines. Paradoxically, even with osteoporosis, the body can still be short of calcium in a form it can use.

Chronic inflamation

Excess acids within the body attack the tissues and organs, resulting in chronic inflammation. The reverse holds true as well in that chronic inflammation, when it occurs for whatever reason, will make the body acidic. The skin and kidneys are especially sensitive to the harmful acids. Skin rashes, eczema, blotching and itching can occur and the kidneys can become inflamed, which can lead to frequent urinary tract infections.

In a state of acidosis, there is less oxygen available to the body which makes the body more conducive for anaerobic bacteria to get a foothold and cancer to start. It is the anaerobic bacteria that are found in root-filled teeth and cavitation infections, and the toxins they produce, that are a major source of MCD. Acid buildup also affects the body's immune function by seriously diminishing the production of white blood cells. Not only are there fewer white blood cells, but those that are produced are not as effective, which makes it even easier for infection to take hold.

Chronic inflammation on its own causes an increase in acidity, so infections, cavitations and root fillings not only have toxins from bacteria creating acid conditions by themselves, they also create chronic inflammation which in turn increases the acid environment. A vicious circle is created that feeds on itself becoming ever more dangerous to health over time.

THE LATER STAGES OF ACIDITY

As time goes on, the acids build up in the organs where they begin to disrupt normal functioning. Without restoring pH balance, the lipids in the cell walls cause them to harden and solidify. The organs deteriorate as the cells die off, which further exacerbate the acidic condition. Now the body's state of acidosis is a prime breeding ground for pathogens such as bacteria, fungi, molds and parasites, which feed off of the diseased tissues and organs. Acidosis literally destroys the body from the inside out, paving the way for disease to take over.

MONITORING pH

Great attention must be paid to pH. A century ago, diet alone could influence pH to such a degree that it could be brought back into normal limits. Unfortunately, this is no longer the case mainly due to the reduced quality of food and the poor response of an increasingly toxic population.

Saliva and Urine pH Graph

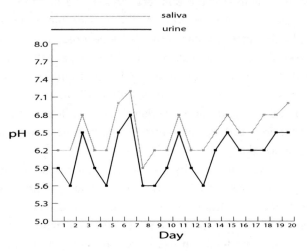

Fig. 2.1 The pH of the urine and saliva of a healthy individual against time. The levels are a little too low but not bad in this day and age.

Saliva and Urine pH Graph

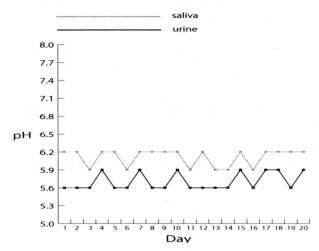

Fig. 2.2 The pH of someone under toxic load in an acidic state.

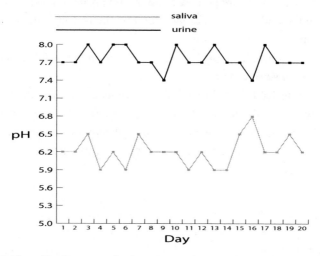

Fig. 2.3 The pH of urine is higher than saliva. Correcting cases like this takes the longest time. We believe this is due to deep-seated infections; mainly viral.

SUMMARY

- Toxins are absorbed from the environment in food, air, water, medications, recreational drugs, and personal and household products.
- Toxins are also produced by anaerobic bacteria from focal infections such as cavitation infections and root-filled teeth.
- Dental treatment can be a major source of metal, chemical and infective toxins.
- The quantity of toxin has no bearing on where the symptoms are, the severity of the symptoms or what symptoms manifest.
- Toxins reduce cell metabolism, i.e. the efficiency of the cell to function properly.
- Toxins have a greater effect on a nutritionally compromised body and by their own action can reduce the availability of vital nutrients.

- Modern diets are generally poor, and prone to produce acidosis in the body. This is compounded by the action of the toxins and chronic inflammation.
- The alteration of pH has a huge effect on the health and healing response of a patient.
- Toxins lead to acidity, which in turn lead to a weakened immune system and a lower utilisation of oxygen at a cellular level.
- *Toxins, acidity, a weak immune system and a lack of oxygen* to the cells have to be corrected or eliminated for any MCD to resolve.

3 DENTAL TOXINS EXPLAINED

This chapter will give more details about the type and danger of toxins in dental treatment with reference to medical treatment as well. This will be dealt with by a section on dental materials such as mercury amalgam and other metals and chemicals used; and the methods of dental treatment which can influence toxicity problems such as focal infections from cavitations, extractions, root fillings and gum disease. The choice of materials to be used in any dental treatment is discussed in the next chapter.

DENTAL MATERIALS

To fill decayed teeth, dentists use one or more of the following materials:

- **Amalgam** – a mixture of mercury, silver, tin, copper and trace elements. Poor aesthetics restrict the use of amalgam to posterior (back) teeth.
- **Metal alloys** – nowadays nickel, chrome, palladium, silver, copper and tantalum are the most used metals with gold, platinum and titanium less often used. In the past, gold alloys were the most often used. All metals in dentistry are alloys, i.e. mixtures of metals, usually between five and seven. These alloys are used for bridges, crowns, inlays, onlays and sometimes dentures. Some alloys can have porcelain or ceramic fused to them for aesthetics in what is called a bonded or VMK crown.
- **Composites** – petroleum-based plastic materials. They can be used for simple fillings directly in the mouth and hardened with

a special light or made into crowns and inlays and stuck into the teeth with composite cement. Composites contain and release a substance called BIS-GMA, which can cause problems.

- **Ceramics** – aesthetically excellent, but have to be made in a laboratory. They are used for small bridges and crowns as well as inlays. Certain ceramics can be cut out of a block by the dentist so no laboratory is involved. There are at present issues with aesthetics and fit with these blocks which are likely to be resolved within a few years.

- **Zirconium** – used for crowns and bridges. It is very hard and bright white. It is cut from a block in the laboratory and covered with ceramic for better aesthetics. Some zirconium techniques rely on old fashioned acidic cements to keep it in place in the mouth and the aesthetics are not as good as pure ceramic used alone. Some types of composite BIS-GMA containing cements can be used with zirconium. Pure ceramic is fairly weak and can break, whereas zirconium is very strong.

- **Glass-ionomers and compomers** – used for less permanent fillings, usually in children only, as they have a tendency to dissolve.

- **Cements** – used to stick the repairs in place. There are many types of cement: some are acidic, some containing formaldehyde, others are more benign.

- **Local anaesthetics** – used to numb up the teeth giving the characteristic fat face feeling. Most anaesthetics are made from coal tar derivatives and break down in the liver to aniline dyes which theoretically increases the risk of cancer. The risk of cancer from dental aniline anaesthetics has never been quantified. Hopefully it is a small risk over a lifetime, but no-one really knows. Happily, some anaesthetics do not break down into aniline dyes, for to undergo dental treatment without anaesthesia is impossible for most people.

- **Topical fluoride** – Prevents tooth decay, but is a grade 2 poison. Diet and good oral hygiene are more important factors.

- **Toothpaste** – helps in getting teeth clean, but not essential. Read the labels carefully when choosing toothpaste. Find one that does not contain fluoride, sodium laurel sulphate, sugar (in various guises) and artificial colours and flavourings.

- **Bleaching** – considered safe to use as long as the bleach is mild and there is no metal in the mouth.

DENTAL MATERIAL TOXICITY

All materials have a toxic potential, some a lot worse than others. Let us start with the worst offender – silver amalgam, or more correctly – mercury amalgam.

Amalgam

There is a huge body of literature published about the detrimental effects of mercury amalgam fillings. What is written here is about 0.5% of what is available. This book is not intended as a definitive work on the pathology of amalgam. It will demonstrate that amalgam affects health, and how it does it. For more detailed information, see the resource section at the website: *www.toxicdentistryexposed.com*.

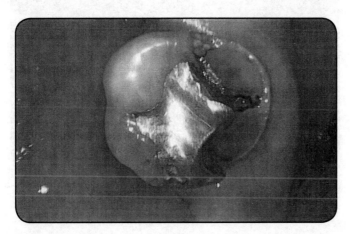

Fig. 3.1 This is a typical amalgam filling that has expanded with age and cracked the tooth. The filling has stayed in place, but it has expanded forcing one complete side of the tooth to break off.

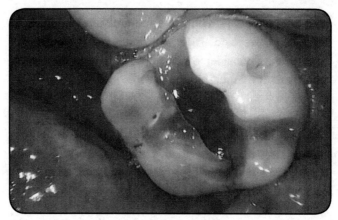

Fig. 3.2 Cracks in a tooth from an amalgam filling.

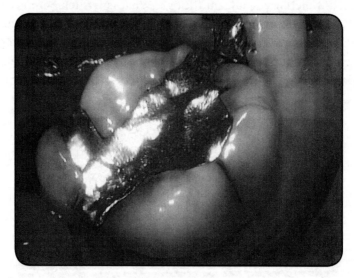

Fig. 3.3 A crack down the side of a tooth due to the expansion of the amalgam filling.

At present all the major dental authorities support the use of amalgam. Hopefully this will change soon. After all, it has only been shown scientifically to be detrimental to human health since 1927 by Dr Stock. Mercury amalgam is the most commonly used dental filling material and has been so for nearly 200 years. Amalgam is a mixture

38

of 50% mercury and the other 50% being tin, silver, and copper with a few trace elements depending on the manufacturer. The mercury content of the filling is not stable and leaks out constantly 24 hrs a day, especially after eating, drinking hot drinks and brushing teeth. Mercury is one of the most toxic metals naturally occurring on the planet and significantly is a known potent neurotoxin. Mercury damages nerve and brain tissue.

There are no minimum thresholds for the toxic effects of mercury. This means that it causes damage at all concentrations no matter how small. Mercury comes off amalgam as vapour throughout the entire life of the filling (see *Fig. 3.4*, page 39).

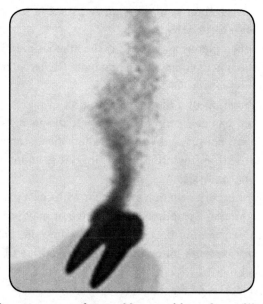

Fig. 3.4 Mercury vapour from a 22-year-old amalgam filling after being rubbed by an eraser. (Courtesy of *www.IAOMT.org*).

This vapour goes into the lungs, which have no defence mechanisms against mercury, and within seconds, the mercury is deposited in the brain and all vital organs. This is what the amalgam manufacturers say about *their own* products:

The use of amalgam is contraindicated in:
- contact to dissimilar metal restorations;
- patients with severe renal deficiency;
- patients with known allergy to amalgam;
- for retrograde or endodontic fillings (root fillings or root canals);
- under a cast crown (metal crown or metal-ceramic crown);
- in children under 6 and;
- in expectant mothers.

Side-effects:
- This product contains mercury that is known to cause birth defects.
- Lichen planus may form on the mucous membrane which is in contact with amalgam (lichen planus is a pre-cancerous condition).
- Inhalation of a high concentration of mercury vapour can cause almost immediate dyspnea, cough, fever, nausea and vomiting, diarrhoea, stomatitis, salivation, metallic taste, gingivitis, and cardiac abnormalities.
- Respiratory irritation may occur with chest pain and tightness. Symptoms may resolve or may progress to necrotising bronchiolitis, pneumonia, pulmonary oedema, pneumothorax, interstitial fibrosis and **death.**
- Acidosis and renal damage may also occur. *(G M-H: Remember the importance of pH regulation!)*
- Allergy reactions that may occur in previously exposed persons include dermatitis, encephalitis and **death.**
- Metal fume fever, an influenza-like illness, may occur due to inhalation of freshly formed metal oxide particles. Symptoms may be delayed 4 to 12 hours

and begin with sudden onset of thirst, a metallic taste in the mouth, dryness of mucous membranes, lassitude and a general feeling of malaise. Also, fever, chills, muscular pain, mild to severe headaches, nausea, profuse sweating, excessive urination, diarrhoea and prostration can occur.

- Chronic inhalation is characterised by fine tremors and erethism. Tremors first affect the hand, then become evident in the face, arms and legs. Erethism is manifested by abnormal shyness, blushing, self-consciousness, depression or despondency, resentment of criticism, irritability or excitability, headache, fatigue and insomnia. In severe cases, hallucinations, loss of memory, and mental deterioration may occur. Concentrations as low as 0.03mg/m3 (30ppm) have induced psychiatric symptoms in humans. *(G M-H: Chronic inhalation of mercury is what all amalgam wearers incur.)*
- Other effects may include salivation, gingivitis, stomatitis, loosening of teeth, blue lines of the gums, diarrhoea, chronic pneumonitis and mild anaemia.
- Tremors and involuntary movements can occur in babies still in the womb. Mercury is excreted in breast milk.
- Paternal reproductive effects and effects on fertility have been reported in male rats following repeated inhalation exposures.

When placing or removing amalgam fillings:
- protective gloves must be worn;
- safety goggles must be worn;
- appropriate protective clothing must be worn and;
- exhaust or general dilution ventilation must be employed to meet permissible exposure limits.

41

These are **not our words**; they are written by the amalgam producers about amalgam and included in the packs sold to dentists.

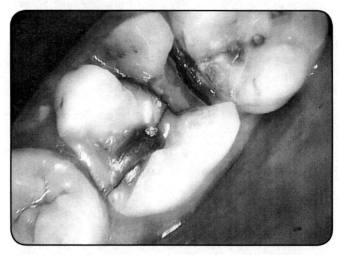

Fig. 3.5 These are cracks made by amalgam expanding as it corrodes. All amalgam fillings expand; all amalgam-filled teeth are cracked; no exception. This tooth still tests 'alive' but what are its chances long-term? Poor.

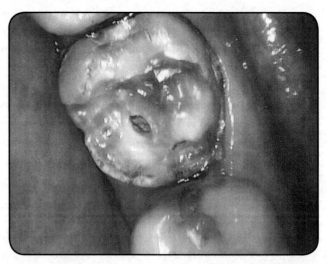

Fig. 3.6 The tooth has died due to the injury to the nerve when the amalgam was placed.

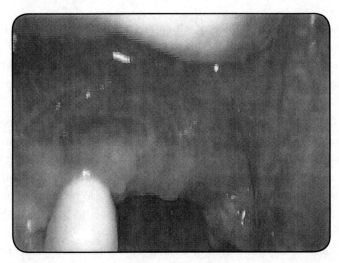

Fig. 3.7 This is a typical amalgam tattoo. Surgical removal of this tattoo gave the patient significant health improvements.

An amalgam tattoo is a discolouration of the gum area due to the different metals of an amalgam filling corroding and being deposited in the gum.

Analysis of a typical amalgam tattoo	
Silver	466000mcg/kilo
Mercury	7470mcg/kilo

These values are over 100 times higher than normal tissue would be. Metal ions build up in the gum; this is seen in the dark lines around crowned teeth and in the dark 'amalgam tattoos'. Analysis of these tattoos shows remarkably high concentrations of all types of metal ions; we know, we have done the analysis.

There is absolutely no logical reason why such a toxic material should be still in use. Mr average dentist is less culpable in this mat-

43

ter than organised dentistry which has resolutely supported the use of amalgam, despite all the massive amounts of scientific knowledge demonstrating the harm amalgam can do. Why do dentists, or more accurately, the dental organisations like the British Dental Association (BDA) and American Dental Association (ADA), continue to ignore the increasing clamour from the lay and scientific community about amalgam? Primarily for two reasons: Firstly, fear of the consequences of admitting amalgam is dangerous to health. After promoting its use and safety for years against overwhelming evidence, the dentists do not want to be held responsible for the damage to people's health they are directly guilty of causing. Secondly, they do not see the havoc wrought by amalgam on health.

Sick patients go to their medical doctor not back to the dentist, and few medical doctors ask about amalgam. Furthermore, the onset of a problem caused by amalgam may be years after the initial exposure to it and no correlation is made between the mercury fillings and the symptoms displayed by the patient.

NEUROLOGICAL CONDITIONS

Mercury destroys the blood brain barrier allowing different molecules into the brain which should never be there. In multiple sclerosis (MS) and Parkinson's, increased mercury levels have been noted in the cerebrospinal fluid (CSF).

The Autism Research Institute is convinced that mercury is the prime cause of autism and related syndromes. ARI has published a 70-page web document called *Autism: A Unique Type of Mercury Poisoning*. In brief they state: 'The similarities between the symptoms of mercury toxicity and autism, considering the exposure to mercury of the foetus and child, suggest that autism is a form of mercury poisoning.'

Indeed, if mercury is chelated from the body, autistic symptoms can be markedly reduced, which is an excellent indicator that ARI are right in their accusation against mercury. Prof Boyd Haley has shown that autistic children lack the mechanism for excreting mercury and that the hormone oestrogen is protective against this toxic substance. This is why boys are more likely to be affected than girls. Mercury containing vaccines deliver a dose of mercury 64 times an adult-allowed exposure, so with multiple vaccines from birth, mother's mercury from her amalgam fillings passing through the umbilical cord delivered to the developing baby, and mercury concentrated in the breast milk, the epidemic of autism now being experienced can be explained.

Psychosis and other effects

In this area there has been much misdiagnosis due to the fact that the medical doctors were, and are, unaware of the release of mercury from a patient's fillings. Psychiatric disturbances have been seen in 12-year-old children due to mercury. One paediatrician told me, 'No-one would ever be stupid enough to use mercury in fillings. I am glad I have the silver ones'. Oh dear! Anxiety and depression have been reduced by selenium, the symptoms coming back when the selenium supplement was stopped. The supplementation of selenium reduces the amount of mercury available in the body, so as the levels of mercury fell in the body, so did the level of symptoms. The lower the levels of selenium, the more anxiety and depression were experienced.

Patients with mercury in the brain at low chronic, so-called sub-toxic levels, were compared to patients without mercury. The mercury patients had short-term memory problems, obsessive-compulsive behaviour, and increased anxiety and psychotism. Apart from this, they were entirely normal! Permanent neuromuscular changes have been noted on workers exposed to inorganic mercury. Common misdiagnoses of mercury posioning are neurasthenia, hysteria and schizophrenia. Other symptoms include tremor, memory loss, eye problems, mood change, decreased self-confidence, increased sweating, and sleep disturbances. Inability to comprehend or accept new ideas is another feature of mercury exposure at low levels.

Obsessive-compulsive behaviour, such as the constant washing of hands, turning around 10 times before entering a shower, constant repetition of conversations, etc. is very often associated with mercury exposure from amalgam fillings. Sometimes the illogical behaviour is recognized by the patient, but even so, it cannot be altered. In tests, dentists who worked with mercury showed reduced hand co-ordination,

45

concentration and memory when compared to a similar group of *dentists who did not work with mercury*. The longer the dentists had worked with mercury, the greater were the effects. The average was a 13.9% reduction. Intelligence was reduced as well in the dentist, which may explain a lot.

Mercury and Alzheimer's

Twenty percent of the population in England over 80 years old has Alzheimer's. This disease was first described in 1907, it is, therefore, a new disease. High levels of mercury are deposited in Alzheimer's brains; these levels of mercury being more out of balance than any other trace element. The early theories of aluminium being a cause have been abandoned after finding that the tissue samples where contaminated by the sampling instruments.

Rats given mercury show the same irreversible changes in their brains as happens in human brains. Amalgam is considered a likely source of this damaging mercury.

A successful way of helping Alzheimer's victims is to give them acetyl-L-carnitine: a compound made in the body. The body needs methionine to make carnitine, and mercury reduces the amount of methionine available to the body. All the research neatly fits together. The age of onset of this disease is reducing; cases have been reported of patients in their thirties starting to get Alzheimer's symptoms.

INTERESTING MERCURY–ALZHEIMER'S FACTS

- Mercury vapour inhaled in quantities similar to what people with amalgam fillings inhale, gives rats and monkeys the same brain lesions as seen in Alzheimer's brains.
- Mercury causes irreversible brain tangles in rats similar to the brain tangles seen in Alzheimer's brains.
- Mercury in Alzheimer's brains is significantly higher than in normal brains.
- Alzheimer's patients have twice as much mercury in the blood than control patients.
- Very low levels of mercury can cause the amyloid plaques in brains, like the plaques of Alzheimer's brain.

46

- There is a certain genotype that predisposes you to acquiring Alzheimer's. This is the APO4 genotype. Those fortunate enough to have the APO1 genotype do not get Alzheimer's. The difference between these two genotypes is that the APO4 gene has two arginine aminoacids and the APO1 has two cysteine aminoacids. Cysteine gives you protection from mercury, whereas arginine does not. APO2 and APO3 genotypes have one arginine and one cysteine; people with these genes get Alzheimer's, but not at the rate of those with the APO4 genes. This is again clear evidence of the mercury–Alzheimer's connection.
- Prof Boyd Haley, Univ. of Kentucky states quite firmly, 'Mercury poisoning bears all the diagnostic hallmarks of Alzheimer's disease.'

What all this means in plain English is that we are 99.9% sure that mercury causes Alzheimer's, but until we can experiment on live humans, we cannot prove it 100%. Obviously live human experimentation is unethical except it seems for the American Dental Association's experiments on Portuguese orphans, so common sense should prevail and the use of mercury in filling materials be stopped.

MERCURY AND CHILDREN

Animal and human experiments show that mercury from the mother's amalgam fillings are stored in the foetus and concentrated in the mother's milk after birth. If the mother drinks alcohol during pregnancy, the amount of mercury deposited in the foetus increases. Mercury from the mother's amalgam fillings can decrease a child's intelligence, reduce his or her learning capacity and make them hyperactive.

MERCURY AND BACTERIA

Mercury from dental amalgam enters the gut and one of the effects is to cause some of the gut bacteria to become antibiotic resistant. These antibiotic resistant bacteria pass on their resistance, not just to their offspring, but to bacteria from other species. Antibiotic resistant bacteria is an ever increasing problem.

Of all the metals in amalgam: mercury, silver, tin and copper, mercury is the largest problem. However, silver and tin are also released and can act as toxins in the body. Mercury is released as a vapour and is far and away the main culprit in damage to health from amalgam fillings.

Dental metals

Dental metal alloys are used in crowns, bridges, inlays, some dentures and implants. Metals are always used in combination, never alone. These combinations are called alloys. Typically, a dental metal alloy will contain from 5 to 7 different metals.

Virtually all known metals have been used in dentistry; in the past, it was mainly gold, silver, platinum, palladium, and copper; today it is more likely to be nickel, chrome and titanium because they are less expensive. Not so long ago, beryllium-containing alloys were in common usage. Beryllium is a potent cancer causing metal; so is nickel, which is also behind many allergic reactions. Beryllium is fortunately no longer used, but nickel is still in common use.

DENTAL METALS AND CORROSION

> 'Dissimilar metals in a moist environment will release the least precious metal.'
>
> Faraday's Law

There are over 1000 different alloys on the market without any safety tests ever being performed on them, either individually or when used together. These alloys will corrode in the mouth releasing metals into the body.

If fillings and crowns are done at different times or by different dentists, the probability is that the alloys used are not the same. Different alloys together in the mouth will corrode, releasing metal ions: Faraday's Law.

Even if only one alloy is used, corrosion stills take place. This is because when the alloy is cast in the laboratory, the different metals in the alloy are not evenly mixed. There is always more of one

48

metal at one end of the casting than at the other end. This difference in concentrations of metal will cause corrosion and metal ion release even within a single casting.

Amalgam and metal alloys in the mouth together cause up to *10 times* more mercury to be released into the body than if amalgam was alone in the mouth. Even worse is an alloy on top of an amalgam filling, as this drives the mercury through the nerves of the teeth directly into the brain.

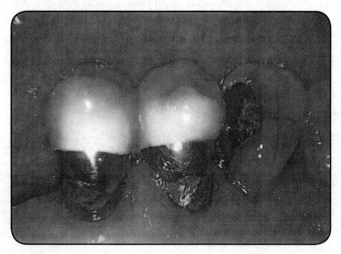

Fig. 3.8 Amalgam 'patches' at the base of a metal crown. This is the worst possible scenario for corrosion and mercury release.

Also remember that only amalgam produces mercury vapour, which is why it is the most dangerous of all metals used in dentistry.

ALLERGIES AND DENTAL METALS

Nickel is carcinogenic and allergenic; gold reduces immune function, hence gold injections for arthritis. Titanium gathers in the spleen. All metals have a dark side to their character. Sensitivity to metals can be tested using a MELISA test. This will show if a patient has an allergic response to a metal, but will not show if the patient is being poisoned by the metal.

49

Dental metals are either in the teeth or in the jawbone. You are exposed to them 24 hours a day every day of the year. This constant exposure can cause allergy or sensitivity to build up over time. So if you have never been exposed to titanium, for instance, you may test as okay for this metal. In a few years time, however, after constant exposure to the metal, an allergy or sensitivity may occur. If allergy or sensitivity occurs, for your health's sake, the metal needs to be removed. So perhaps a non-metal solution is preferable in the first instance. As a very general rule of thumb, if there are any symptoms causing concern, do not have metal restorations at all. After all, 'Only robots should have metal spare parts.' Prof Vera Stejskal, inventor of the MELISA test.

If you are in perfect health and insist on having metal teeth, at the very least get tested beforehand to see if you have any sensitivity to the metals that are to be used.

> **Caution:** Before having any work done, read the treatment section. Do not rush into treatment. Successful treatment is like a ballroom dance: to be effective it has to be done in sequence, each step following the other. Failure to follow the sequence can make a bad situation a lot worse.

Composites

Composites are a mixture of ceramic particles and plastic. There are nanocomposites, hybrid composites, fluid composites, light setting composites, chemical setting composites, dual setting composites and so on. All are basically the same: ceramic particles in plastic. The shades available for composites are many, and for an aesthetic filling they can be accurately matched to the shade of the teeth. The shades are different metal oxides. It is possible to obtain composites with no metal oxides, however, metal oxides are not pure metals and react quite differently. Our experience is that for the great majority, but not all, of patients, metal oxides are not a problem. The same can be said for the aluminium content of composites. Composites which are fully cured give off little aluminium. A composite which is not fully cured or set will release aluminium, but again not in vast amounts. To put this in perspective, anyone who drinks a can of any fizzy drink will ingest from that one can many times more, 100 fold at least, of aluminium than any composite filling could emit.

BIS-BMA, EDT-GMA and camphor-quinines

The toxicity problems associated with composites are due to the BIS-GMA (bisphenol A glycidyl methacrylate) phase of the plastic and the photo-initiators (camphor quinones). Both these types of chemicals can cause reactions in the sensitive patient. It is rare, but does occasionally happen. Oestrogen formation and release as well as formaldehyde release has been laid at the door of BIS-GMA. Whether the amounts released are significant to the general population is unknown, but sensitive patients can react to composite. We were concerned about this, but we found that if a composite was fully set, then polished, then washed thoroughly, BIS-GMA was very seldom detectable. Symptoms such as rashes anywhere in the body, burning and itching sensation locally, even pressure pain are symptoms we have noticed. BIS-GMAs are the subject of ongoing research (see *www.IAOMT.org* for the latest news on this subject).

One particular composite is based on fibreglass. Some patients who are sensitive to conventional composites tolerate the fibreglass composite, but not all do. Some patients are sensitive to the fibreglass composite, but can tolerate the conventional composite. There have been non-BIS-GMA composites developed in the past, but unfortunately the manufacturers have abandoned these and they are no longer generally available.

Acrylics or plastics

Acrylics are used in dentures. Usually the teeth and the base are acrylic. The teeth are not the problem, it is the base. The base is made from a powder and liquid monomer. It is the monomer that causes the reactions. Usually, these are localised to burning mouth syndrome and the like. Reaction to monomers is more common than it is given credit for, but the problems appear to be localised in most cases, not systemic.

51

Occasionally, we have seen reaction to the colouring content of acrylics: the pink colour in the denture base. The answer to this is to use a clear acrylic with no colouring component. Aesthetics may be compromised, but not health. Nylon-based materials are coming to the fore now, replacing in some part the traditional use of acrylics in the making of dentures. From a toxicity viewpoint they are excellent, as the polymers that make them up are very long chained and do not appear to give off any reactive substances. From a comfort viewpoint they are excellent as well as they are flexible rather than hard, which makes them significantly easier to tolerate than acrylic dentures.

It is not all positive, however; there are some technical features that limit their usefulness. For instance, it is sometimes impossible to add a tooth after a fresh extraction to a nylon-based denture; the denture must be scrapped and a new one made. The aesthetics can be compromised as well, as there is sometimes a thin clasp at the neck of a tooth to hold the nylon denture in place. The colour of the nylon dentures is either clear or various shades of pink and occasionally this pink clasp can be visible. By and large, this is a small price to pay for the other advantages of the material.

Ceramics, zirconium and CAD/CAM restorations

Zirconium is covered by ceramic; so what applies to ceramic applies to zirconium. Ceramic crowns not fired correctly in the oven at a high enough temperature or for too short a time, can release aluminium. This cannot be detected easily. One can hope that the dental technician firing the ceramic is competent and the vast majority of dental technicians are thoroughly competent. Whether this is a problem in the real world is not known. Overall we would doubt that there is a significant problem with this. The problems with these types of restorations tend to be more the method of preparation of the teeth, the toxicity of the cements used to stick them in place, and the wear on opposing teeth rather than an overt toxic release from the ceramic material. Also, the rigidity of ceramic compares unfavourably to the slight 'give' of composite, and ceramics transmit more temperature change through to the tooth than do composite materials. Both these traits can be a problem for ceramic restorations, but they are not directly toxicity problems.

Computer-cut crowns and inlays (CAD/CAM restorations) can have ceramic added. They can be used without any ceramic additions as well. The composition of the blocks of material from which the crowns and inlays are cut can be considered for all intents and purposes to be the same as ceramic. In the real world, there appear to be very few patients who react to these materials. Once again, it is the cement holding them in place that is the problem.

Cements, glas-ionomers and compomers

Cements come in a variety of forms. There are composite cements, zinc cements, polycarbonate cements and so on and so forth. All types of cement usually, but not invariably, contain fluoride which is released slowly, supposedly reducing the risk of caries. All cements either release BIS-GMA or other chemicals into the body or are acidic.

TECHNICAL ISSUES

More patients react to the cement than to the filling it is sticking in place. Dental cement toxicity is complex due to the number of different types of cement that are available. As a general rule, the older types of cement cause less problems of a systemic nature than the newer types of cement, but the older type of cements are more acidic and can cause teeth to become sensitive or even die. Glas-ionomers and compomers all contain fluoride and all are mildly acidic. These are often used as filling materials in their own right for children's teeth.

LEAKAGE AND DECAY

Another major problem with cement is its solubility. They all can slowly dissolve away with time; although, it isn't as much of a problem with composite types of cement. This can lead to the filling or restoration leaking and decay starting under the filling. This is less of a problem than it would seem in the real world. Quite often when fillings are removed, the same goes for crowns etc., it is obvious that there has been leakage due to staining of the tooth, but no decay can be seen. This can be attributed to the toxic nature of metal restorations inhibiting, for a while at least, the bacterial growth necessary for decay to start and also is a reflection on the diet of the patient. The length of time the leakage has been there and the type of diet plays a significant role. All such gaps between restorations and teeth must be dealt with as it is only a matter of time before decay sets in. With composite fillings such decay can start very rapidly indeed.

Topical fluorides

Fluoride gels are applied to teeth to prevent decay or caries. They are effective in some measure as they poison the bacteria that cause decay. One could use arsenic gels to the same effect, but there might be a problem with public acceptance of arsenic. Fluoride applied in a gel is supposed to change the chemical nature of the tooth enamel and make it more resistant to decay. This is somewhat questionable. However, painting a child's teeth with a class 2 registered poison: fluoride, reduces the decay rate. We doubt whether this is a sensible policy as a sensible diet and good dental hygiene are the most important factors in reducing decay.

HYDROFLUORIC ACID

A small amount of all fluoride gels on teeth will be swallowed. Fluoride in the stomach reacts with the hydrochloric acid of the stomach and produces hydrofluoric acid. This particular acid is so strong it will dissolve glass. Only small amounts of hydrofluoric acid are made, but the fact that it is formed at all must be detrimental to the child. Similarly, the fluoride in drinking water will produce hydrofluoric acid in the gut as will swallowed fluoride toothpaste. We think that hydrofluoric acid formation is why stomach pains in children are more prevalent in fluoridated areas than clean water areas, but that is our observation only. From a personal perspective, we would suggest that even small amounts of hydrofluoric acid in the stomach cannot be positive. Adding fluoride to the water to prevent tooth decay is as nonsensical as adding sunblock to the water to prevent sunburn. Both only work when applied topically, i.e. rubbed on, not systemically when swallowed.

The fluoride added to the water also causes the increased absorption of lead, especially in certain ethnic groups. In fluoridated areas, this is seen in increased crime and vandalism rates within these ethnic groups. It must be considered a form of racism.

TOOTHPASTES

Fluoride toothpastes are poisonous. There is enough fluoride in a tube of toothpaste to kill a seven-year-old child. Every year, there are 'incidents' involving small children swallowing fluoridated toothpastes, some ending in the death of the child. Another constituent of toothpastes is sodium laurel sulphate. This is a foaming agent, which is why you look like a rabid dog when you use these toothpastes. Sodium laurel sulphate is a detergent; a lot is known about its detrimental effects on health. Sugar is a common ingredient of toothpaste, like sorbitol. Difficult though that might be to understand why a supposedly decay-producing agent is put into toothpaste, a nice sweet taste sells well and sales are more important than health to the manufacturer. Sugar is cheap and acts as a binder too. Artificial colourings and flavourings abound for aesthetic and taste reasons; they play no part in the cleaning of teeth. The only role they play is to increase the 'attractiveness' of the product to the consumer.

Toothpaste is not essential in getting teeth clean. It helps, but it is not really necessary. A good cleaning technique with a properly-shaped toothbrush or ultrasound brush is the vital factor. We are all conditioned into using toothpaste like Pavlov's dogs. When we pick up a toothbrush we automatically want to put toothpaste on it. The function of toothpaste is mild abrasion to help remove the dental plaque or film that sticks to the teeth. If the toothpaste is too abrasive it will wear your teeth away; smokers toothpastes fit into this category. Cosmetic toothpastes contain mild bleaching agents in the hope of making teeth whiter. The old cosmetic toothpastes which stained the gums red in order to make the teeth whiter are no longer available as the dye used to stain the gums was carcinogenic. Read the labels carefully when choosing toothpaste. Find one that does not contain fluoride, sodium laurel sulphate, sugar (in various guises) and artificial colours and flavourings.

Bleaching

The fashion of bleaching teeth is presently in vogue. Teeth do discolour with age. Staining builds up inside the actual tooth structure; this is called an intrinsic stain. An extrinsic stain is just on the outside surface of the teeth and can be polished away. Smoking makes things worse as the smoke is over 600°C and can damage the enamel allowing nicotine to stain the teeth brown. Smoking creates intrinsic and extrinsic stains on and in teeth.

HYDROGEN PEROXIDE

Bleach applied to teeth is detectable in the blood within less than one minute after application. This does not on the face of it sound too positive, but your white cells actually collect bacteria inside of themselves and make their own bleach to kill the bacteria. They kill themselves at the same time. There is a therapy that injects hydrogen peroxide directly into the veins in order to oxygenate the body. Whether the small amount of bleach found in the blood after teeth bleaching is harmful is doubtful considering the amount injected into the body with hydrogen peroxide therapy, but once again, no-one really knows.

DESICCATING BLEACHING

Bleach that is applied for too long at a high concentration under high temperature, desiccates or dries up the teeth producing minute stress cracks in the enamel. This gives the bright white uniform 'television newsreader' look so popular nowadays. It looks artificial because that is exactly what it is: artificial. Real teeth are not uniform in colour individually, neither are all exactly the same shade. Desiccating bleaching creates this uniformity. When the enamel repairs itself the brightness fades so more bleach has to be applied. The long-term effects of repeated desiccating bleaching are not known, but it is not likely to be positive. The bleaching lamps and other bleaching gadgets are just marketing tools to make the bleaching appear more technical and complicated. All they do is raise the temperature to make the bleach work quicker.

The toxicity problem with bleaching occurs when bleach is applied to metal restorations, especially amalgam. The bleaching agent, hydrogen peroxide, is very chemically active and easily breaks down to water and oxygen. The oxygen reacts strongly with amalgam releasing large amounts of mercury. We would not recommend bleaching for anyone with any metal in their mouth; certainly not if they have amalgam fillings.

This is not to say bleaching is all bad. Mild bleaching agents applied at the correct concentrations over some weeks at home do penetrate the teeth and remove the intrinsic stains. They bring the teeth back to their original shade and the look is natural. Fillings stay the same colour and do not become whiter; a fact to be borne in mind when contemplating bleaching. Bleaching can make the teeth more reactive to hot and cold and we have experienced heart rate increases and transient tachycardia (accelerated heart rate) on the more sensitive patients. If you are considering having your teeth bleached, make sure no metals are present in the teeth and that a mild bleach is used at the dentists. At home, you can continue to use the bleach every other day until you achieve the desired colour. This method usually does not require top-ups of bleach for several years.

Root-canal-filling materials

The purpose of root-canal-filling materials is to fill the space inside the tooth where a nerve used to be and to prevent or actively kill bacteria inside of the root canal chamber. No root-canal-filling material can do any of these things effectively. The health disaster that root canals can cause is dealt with later on. Root-canal-treated teeth or dead teeth are centres of chronic inflammation and infection. The toxins produced by these inflammations and infections can have systemic effects anywhere in the body. The trouble caused by such infections is out of all proportion to the amount of toxin released.

This section will deal with the toxicity issues of some of the root-canal-filling materials. The materials used in root canals can leak through the tip or apex of the tooth and have direct access to the body. The commonest method of root canal treatment is to put a paste inside the canal and place a thin rod or a point of gutta-percha into the canal. The paste sets and the canal is sealed. At least in theory, but never in practice. Silver rods or points can be used instead of gutta-percha, but this practice is seldom used today. Many years ago, we removed a lower molar tooth that was root-filled and had a silver point poking through the root tip into the bone. The patient had lost the sight of her left eye some six years after the root filling had been done. She recovered the sight of her left eye within two weeks of the removal. This came as a real shock to us at the time.

Paste is usually placed past the tip of the tooth directly into the bone as is the silver or gutta-percha point. Different pastes have different toxicity problems associated with them.

Here is a list of the ingredients and problems of the most commonly used pastes and points:

Root-canal-filling material	Contains
AH26	formaldehyde ammonia bismuth oxide silver

The advice sheet says, 'if swallowed, call a doctor immediately; harmful, irritant. Do not allow undiluted product to reach sewage or ground water.'

Root-canal-filling materials	Contains
Tubli-Seal	4-allyl-2-methoxphenol

58

Pulp Canal Sealer	4-allyl-2-methoxphenol zinc oxide
Sealapex	isobutyl salicylate resin n-ethyl toluene solfonamide resin

The advice sheet says, 'amongst other things, may cause allergic dermatitis and drowsiness, eye and skin irritant.'

DENTAL TREATMENTS THAT CAUSE TOXIC PROBLEMS
Crown and bridges

High-speed drills create tiny microscopic fractures through the teeth. There is a school of thought in Germany that believes bacteria in these cracks are the cause of modern diseases. Whilst this may be a factor, no-one really knows; it is likely to be only part of the problem. In preparing teeth for a crown or a bridge, the enamel is drilled away leaving a tooth stump behind. An impression is taken of the stump and a technician makes a crown to fit onto the stump to look like a new tooth. Any missing teeth either side of the crown can also be replaced this way. This is a called a bridge because it literally bridges the gap. Usually, the teeth either side of the gap are cut down in the same way crowned teeth are and the missing teeth are made of the same material the crowns are and fused to them. Occasionally, it is possible to use just one tooth at the side of the gap as a support, but only in special circumstances.

Infections

Teeth consist of outer enamel, an inner dentine core, and a nerve or pulp in the middle of the tooth. The dentine is a tubular structure with wisps of tissue in each tube connected to the nerve or pulp. There is a constant flow of fluid from the nerve to the dentine and outwards to the enamel. There is also constant exchange of minerals between the enamel and the dentine. This is the ideal situation. Diet can actually reverse this flow and disrupt the mineral exchange, but that is another story. Removing the enamel and making the micro-cracks in the dentine quite often, but not always, damages the inner nerve. The damage can cause the nerve to die slowly over years allowing infection to take hold. This infection can spread from the tooth to the bone and cause acute conditions, pain and abscesses as well as chronic pain-free infections in the tooth and bone. Overheating the tooth during drilling can create the same conditions as well for the nerve or pulp. All infections create toxic load. A dead or infected tooth must be either extracted or root treated. (See pages 82–87 for problems with extractions and root fillings.)

The new way of veneering teeth for aesthetics removes over half of the tooth enamel. This is often done on perfectly healthy teeth. This destruction of enamel for cosmetic reasons may be justified, provided the patient knows the health risk they are running from such destruction. Informed consent as always is vital. In the author's opinion, the greater the amount of enamel left behind after a tooth is prepared for a crown or bridge, the greater the chance of survival for that tooth. We crown teeth but only if no other option is available to us. Crowning should be the last choice in treating a tooth, not the first choice.

Orthodontics

Now to tread on some more professional toes! Orthodontics is the moving of teeth in the jaws to create a good aesthetic result. Moving teeth that end up out of balance with the forces of the muscles of the jaws will inevitably lead to the long-term failure of orthodontic treatment so often experienced by patients.

The overcrowding of teeth seen almost universally on children and adults is a modern phenomenon. It is not seen on skulls until about 200+ years ago. Skulls from the Roman period show beautiful wide dental arches. They did not have the receding chin rat look of today's population. The same development of wide arches can be seen today on those lucky enough to have escaped the ravages of the modern diet. Evolution takes thousands of years to work, not 200 years. The

60

present overcrowded jaws we see are a direct result of modern diet. Weston Price illustrated this in his book *Nutrition and Racial Degeneration* written in the 1930s. What happens is the jaw muscles go into spasm and do not allow the jaw bones to develop. Sugar is the prime culprit for causing jaw muscle spasm. My own daughter ground her baby teeth to the gum line; every night you could hear the grinding. Getting rid of sugar from her diet, albeit with difficulty, stopped her from grinding at night almost immediately. The grinding action is one way muscles show they are in spasm.

ORTHOPAEDIC ORTHODONTICS

The statement 'the teeth are too big for the jaws' is false. It should be 'the jaws are too small for the teeth.' Therefore, extracting teeth to fit the available jaw space is almost always the wrong treatment to do. Occasionally, extracting teeth for orthodontic reasons is justified, but not very often. Expanding the jaw bones to the right size allows the teeth to grow into their rightful places. Sometimes, the teeth will need to be moved, but if the jaw bones are the correct size and in the correct relationship to each other, the teeth usually sort themselves out. This approach is called orthopaedic orthodontics.

Orthopaedic orthodontics measures the skull bones and the size of the teeth. It can then be accurately worked out what the size of the jaw bones should be and their relationship to each other. When the jaw bones are developed, the teeth go into a good aesthetic and functional position in balance between the forces of the tongue from the inside and the lips and cheeks from the outside. The end result is a stable dentition which looks good and functions well with major health benefits to the individual. Patients lucky enough to have had such treatment seldom experience the relapse seen after conventional orthodontic treatment.

ORTHODONTIC EXTRACTION

Orthodontic treatment that extracts teeth can lead to what dentists call collapsed arches. This means that although the teeth may be straight to look at, the fit of the upper teeth against the lower teeth is not in harmony with the shape of the jaw joints and position of the muscles controlling the jaw. The following things can happen.

- Jaw joint trouble (TMD) later on in life.
- Appearance is altered – instead of a wide, pleasing arch form of the mouth, the arches are narrow producing a 'rosebud-shaped' mouth with a weak chin that emphasises the size of the nose.
- Impacted wisdom teeth – lack of development of the jaw bones does not allow room for the wisdom teeth to erupt and they become impacted in the bone.

This is why we have far more wisdom teeth being removed now than ever before.

CASE STUDY 4

Four premolar teeth were extracted when the patient was 13. This has caused the remaining lower back teeth to tilt forwards.

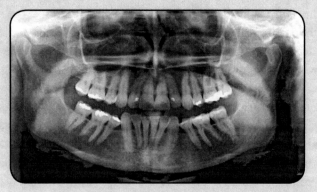

Fig. 3.9 A typical case of orthodontic extraction tilting the teeth in an unnatural direction.

This patient had to have the wisdom teeth removed and had considerable jaw joint trouble as well. This was a direct result of the orthodontic extraction treatment.

Many impacted wisdom teeth have a reduced blood supply and the nerve inside has died. This can lead to infection and cavitation infections both of which have severe toxic consequences.

CASE STUDY 5

We removed two lower impacted wisdom teeth from a 19-year-old girl who had suffered from recurring tonsillitis for several years. The teeth looked normal when removed, no decay or filling in the teeth, and no obvious sign of infection; but when the tooth was cut in half, the nerve (pulp) chamber was empty. The nerve had been dead for a long time.

After extraction, the tonsillitis never returned. The infected teeth were draining back into the tonsil area causing the tonsillitis. The usual treatment of antibiotics only treated the symptoms, but did not address the cause of the tonsillitis.

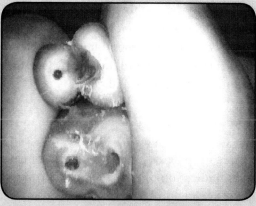

Fig. 3.10 The wisdom tooth cut in half to show the empty pulp chamber.

Another consequence of a lack of jaw bone development is the reduction in maxillary sinus space and the ability to drain. Sinus infections are more frequent and severe as are throat and ear problems. Technically this can be called lack of premaxillary development, and is rampant among today's patients. This in turn increases the probability of allergy problems. So often we have seen allergies and chronic sinus problems resolve when the jaw bone is widened to the correct shape, even in adulthood, especially in conjunction with skilled cranial osteopathy. The effect on children is even more dramatic.

These have been the author's observations over 35 years. Specialist orthodontists would disagree with us. Our reply would be to just take a look with open eyes and mind without trying to protect the status quo.

Failure of diagnosis

Regretfully, many dental remuneration systems are based on the drill, fill and bill basis. The dentist is encouraged to see teeth as individual items that are in need of repair. The tooth repair is done as economically or as cheaply as possible and the insurance, be it private or state funded, foots the bill; sometimes the individual patient pays.

So many patients receive routine dental care that does not address the underlying dental problems. 'Supervised neglect' is the term Dr LD Pankey correctly called this approach. This supervised neglect way of treating dental disease is more expensive in the long-term as it leads to greater dental and general health problems because the underlying problems are not solved. In other words, the patient needs to be examined not just the teeth and gums.

All areas of toxicity must be identified. Whether specific toxins are causing specific problems, is not yet possible to know. Quite often, as patterns of symptoms are recognised, they can be associated with certain types of toxicity. This is not proof of cause and effect, however, just an indication of probability of a connection between the toxin and the symptom. When the toxic load is removed and the symptom also goes, then that is a clear indication that there may well have been a connection between the two. It is still not proof though. For definitive proof of a connection between toxin and symptom, the toxin would need to be replaced and the symptoms return. In real life, this is impossible and certainly would be unethical to do. Know your patient is the mantra as well as know yourself, your strengths and weaknesses. Unless the patient is properly examined, the appropriate treatment may not be done.

Failure to Follow Mechanical Principles

This is about *occlusion* or how the teeth fit against each other and with the jaw joints and muscles. Repairing individual teeth with no regard to the way the tooth functions in relation to the other teeth and jaw structures is often forced on the dentist by the payment schemes and by the lack of knowledge of the dentist as well. Since the basic principles of occlusion where written down in 1927 by Dr Clyde Schyler, there is no need for ignorance in this area. However, it was not taught at my dental school in the 1960s and student dental education does not seem to have improved even now in this regard.

If the teeth are not allowed to function in harmony with the jaw joints and muscles, one of the following will take place.

1. Nothing happens.
2. There is an increased wear on teeth.
3. Fillings and crowns chip and fracture.
4. There is a greater sensitivity to hot and cold on the teeth.
5. Food trapping between teeth increases.
6. The gum recedes from the neck of the tooth.
7. The neck of the tooth becomes thinner: the piezoelectric corrosion of the tooth. This is often confused with an incorrect tooth brushing technique.
8. The bone supporting the teeth is lost (periodontal disease).
9. Overstressed teeth die and need root fillings or extractions.
10. Temporomandibular joint dysfunction syndrome (TMD) can take the form of headaches, fatigue, night grinding, back pain, plus any or all of the above.

So unless the basic mechanical principles of occlusion are known and followed by the dentist, the consequences can be severe for the patient. This is not the place to discuss the various principles of occlusion.

Implants

Now we are treading on feet, not just toes, but we do not mind. It is more important to have truth as your goal than fitting in with the majority. The vast majority of dentists will not appreciate this next section as implants are a major dental source of income. I did my first implant in 1973 and the last one in 1994, so I have considerable experience with them. It took me some time to realise the consequences of what I was doing, as initially the implant seemed to work, but it took several years before any deterioration in health occurred. Connecting the deterioration in health with an implant placed years ago is not easy. Only when the implant is removed and good health restored is the connection made.

THE PROBLEM WITH IMPLANTS

Implants are titanium alloys placed directly into the bone to replace missing teeth. The problem with implants is threefold:

1. Implants are not sealed units; they allow bacteria to proliferate in the joints. In the best case scenario, there is enough space between the various parts of the implant for eight bacteria to fit in line abreast. A tooth has fluid constantly flowing from the tooth neck outwards. This fluid prevents bacteria from penetrating down the root side. Implants have no such fluid protection against bacterial penetration and infection.
2. Quite a lot of the time, they are placed into cavitation infection sites causing the spread of the infection, usually slowly, through the bone.

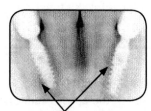

Fig. 3.11 Infected bone around an implant.

66

3. Finally, the crown placed on top of the implant is made from a different alloy than the implant itself. This leads to the inevitable corrosion and release of metals into the body. Few dentists perform any of the tests to see if the mixture of metals they use will affect the health of the patient. They assume, wrongly, that for most patients metals are not a problem. Faraday's Law: dissimilar metals corrode when in contact, works in the mouth as well as in the rest of the known universe. This seems to come as a surprise to some dental schools we have had discussions with. These corrosion metal ions are deposited in the teeth, gums and swallowed into the gut. This corrosion produces electricity which is measurable. This is dental galvanism.

Dental galvanism

The electric potential between teeth and gums due to the release of metal ions by corrosion is what is measured and called the galvanic effect or dental galvanism. Galvanic effects have been used to arrange treatment sequence. The theory goes that the most reactive filling should be removed first and the second most reactive next and so on and that this 'sequential removal' will markedly improve health. The authors did extensive testing in their practice, but found no measurable difference in health benefits if this theory was followed or not. At first glance it is an attractive theory and may have some validity, but in reality it is of no consequence, provided the correct treatment protocols are used as outlined later on. Galvanism only shows that corrosion of the metals in the mouth is taking place and nothing else.

The different electro-potential of the various metals used in dentistry and body piercing has an effect on the nerves. Low electro-potential can stimulate nerve cells, whereas high electro-potential will inhibit nerve transmission. On a significant proportion of patients, this will upset the proprioceptive (internal sensors) feedback loops causing certain muscle groups to be weakened and deteriorate leading to pain, weakness, joint degeneration, even ME. Once again, yet another reason for never using metals in dentistry or in body piercing. The latter seems a very strange practice: to risk ill health for a so-called cosmetic enhancement.

CASE STUDY 6

The symptoms and causes

A lady from Norway had nine implants placed in the preceding three years to replace missing teeth. She did not want to wear dentures. Gradually her health had slipped to such a degree she thought she would be dead within the year. She had a multitude of serious symptoms from allergies, auto-immune conditions to liver and kidney dysfunction. All the symptoms had no known cause despite extensive and expensive testing. An oral surgeon said four of the implants had 'not taken' and should be removed.

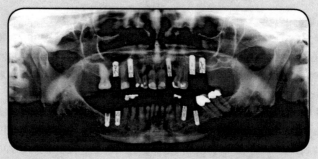

Fig. 3.12 An x-ray of her mouth showing the nine implants.

The treatment

We removed all nine implants under the V-Tox proto-col over two days. The bone around the so-called healthy implants was sent away for toxin analysis to a specialist laboratory in the USA. From the results shown, all the bone was highly toxic. *Fig. 3.13* shows the lab results of the levels of toxicity from the bone around one of the so-called healthy implants. The toxicity in the bone was severe, at the top of the scale used. All five major enzyme systems were inhibited by an average of 90%. No wonder she thought she was dying.

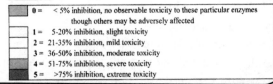

ALT BIOSCIENCE

235 Bolívar Street
Lexington, KY 40508
Phone: (859) 388-9445
FAX: (859) 388-9645
E-mail: info@altcorp.com
www.altbioscience.com

Laboratory Director: Doris Baker, PhD, HCLD, MT
Laboratory Supervisor: Meg Crellin, BS, MT, ASCP
CLIA ID #: 18D0944754

REPORT OF IN VITRO SAMPLE TOXICITY
(Assessed by nucleotide photoaffinity labeling of purified enzymes treated with sample extract)

		Doctor						
		Name:	Dr. Graeme Munro-Hall					
		Address:	Wick End Farm, Wick End					
Sample:	Cavitation Biopsy (Bone)		Stagsden, Bedford MK40 4AF					
	Area # 21		England					
ALT#:	012607-16	Phone:	+44-1234-360793					
Date Sample Analyzed:	1/28/07	FAX:	+44-1234-342793					

Percent Inhibition of Purified Enzyme Activity Relative to a Control with No Extract								
Enzyme Assayed	% Inhibition	Toxicity Level	0	1	2	3	4	5
Phosphorylase Kinase	82.2%	5 = extreme						X
Phosphorylase A	89.4%	5 = extreme						X
Pyruvate Kinase	90.8%	5 = extreme						X
Phosphoglycerate Kinase	88.6%	5 = extreme				.		X
Creatine Kinase	92.4%	5 = extreme						X
Adenylate Kinase	94.0%	5 = extreme						X
Average	90%							X

Toxicity Scale

- **0 =** < 5% inhibition, no observable toxicity to these particular enzymes though others may be adversely affected
- **1 =** 5-20% inhibition, slight toxicity
- **2 =** 21-35% inhibition, mild toxicity
- **3 =** 36-50% inhibition, moderate toxicity
- **4 =** 51-75% inhibition, severe toxicity
- **5 =** >75% inhibition, extreme toxicity

Fig. 3.13 The inhibition of the above tested enzymes was extreme.

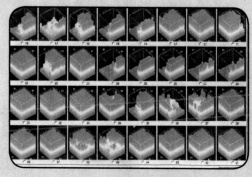

Fig. 3.14 The cavitat scan showed bone infections around all the implants.

The recovery

Testing done at the chairside also showed extreme toxicity around all the implants. After the removal of the implants and the cleaning out of the infections, done correctly, the results were swift and impressive. Within three months the lady was back singing in her church choir and within nine months she was back to her robust health. Re-scanning the area showed full healing of the bone. She gladly wore a partial denture! What is important about this case is:

- How would her doctor connect her implants to her symptoms?
- How would the oral surgeon be able to see toxic bone around the implants?

It is an impossible task for them to do. They did not have the knowledge and experience to connect implants with poor health. If the patient had not done her own research and trusted her instinct that there was something amiss with the implants, her situation would not have improved. Indeed, she thinks she would have been dead within the year. Once again it shows that at some level, the vast majority of patients know where the problems lie.

Case study 7

The symptoms and causes

This case demonstrates the link between toxic dentistry and, what is perceived to be, an unrelated illness. A young man in his early twenties had been diagnosed as paranoid schizophrenic for three years. He had been in and out of various residential establishments since the age of 15. He had one pinhead-sized amalgam in an upper premolar that was put in when he was 14: a year before his mental illness took hold. No treatment tried so far had helped him at all. He was outside society and a burden on it.

He did act very strangely and there was always an undercurrent of potential violence about him. This made working with him particularly stressful for us as we were never sure how controlled he actually was or whether if we turned our backs on him, we would end up with a knife between the shoulder blades! He had no money at all so not only did we not charge him we even ended up paying for his accommodation during his treatment week.

The treatment and recovery

Removing this one amalgam filling and going through the supplementation and vitamin C infusion programme was enough to change his life. He was able to re-enter society, went to university and graduated with a maths degree as well as finding a partner. Far from being a burden on society, he became a contributor instead. He asked for a bill when he left us and paid it all back after some time. This tiny amalgam filling had pressed the button which turned on his mental illness making him hyper-and over-reactive. Removing it correctly had the most profound effect on his life and future.

Focal infections

A focal infection is a persistent bacterial infection limited to a specific organ or region but causing symptoms elsewhere in the body. Conventional dentistry does not accept the fact of focal infection even though doctors and vets do. (It would not be financially advantageous for dentistry to accept it; though of course, this would not be the reason brought forward for its rejection). Focal infection theory was once accepted by dentists, but with the advent of antibiotics the theory fell into disuse.

CHRONIC INFECTIONS

Focal infection is far more fact than theory. Focal infections are for the most part chronic infections. A chronic infection does not have the pain, pus, redness and swelling of an acute infection. It can lie hidden away with no overt symptoms to warn the patient. With chronic infections, the organism wraps a nice protective mucilaginous coat around itself. This coat makes it impervious to the body's natural defences of the immune system. It is in effect 'hidden' from it.

The colony of organisms obtains what it needs from the body: warmth, shelter, food; and dumps the waste products it produces into the body. *Acute* infections we are all familiar with: swelling, redness, increase in temperature and pus formation. These infections are seized on and ruthlessly dealt with by the immune system. Chronic infections protect themselves from this attack. The most frequent area to find these hidden infections are the jaw bones, teeth, tonsils, and maxillary sinuses, in that order, though they can occur in any part of the body. A classic example is the dental cavitation infection. This type of infection has been frequently reported in the literature since 1915 by respected authors such as GV Black and later by Weston Price, but has yet to gain acceptance in the wider dental community.

> 'These infective areas caused problems far greater than could be imagined by their size.'
>
> Dr Weston Price

If it was accepted it would lead to major changes to the usual practice of dentistry, so even though it is 100% proven to be true, the existence of cavitation infections is ignored by the mainstream profession.

THE THEORY OF FOCAL INFECTION

Focal infection was a widely held theory during the first half of the 20th century. It assumed that an infection in one part of the body could cause symptoms in another quite separate area. The way this was supposed to work was that the organisms from the infection site would break away into the blood stream and be carried around in the blood vessels. The blood vessels become steadily narrower and narrower. Artery reduces to arteriole, which in turn reduces to capillary until eventually there is room for just one red blood cell at a time to squeeze through the passage. The invading organism would follow the same route as the blood until it literally became stuck in the ever reducing size of the passages. Wherever this happened, an infection would start in this completely new area of the body. This theory has been revised in the recent past to include the release of toxins: a complex protein mix; which the organisms give off as waste products of their metabolism.

These toxins can be very biologically active and even tiny amounts can have devastating effects on health. Proteins such as 'heat shock 60' emanating from bacteria in the mouth, are now strongly indicated as a cause of heart disease and stroke. The toxins attack injured tissue or tissue weakened by the genetic predisposition of the patient and tissue made vulnerable by inadequate nutrition.

THE COMMON DENTAL SOURCES OF FOCAL INFECTIONS

There are four common sources of focal infections associated with dentistry. These are:
1.   cavitation or NICO infections in bone;
2.   root fillings;
3.   dead and infected teeth;
4.   gum disease.

1. Cavitation or NICO infections in bone
DETECTING CAVITATION INFECTIONS

Cavitation infections, sometimes called Ratner bone lesions, or when causing pain, NICOs (neuralgia-inducing cavitational osteonecrosis), have been reported in the literature for close to 100 years, but have been generally ignored. The reason for this is that they are not easily seen in an x-ray film. The usual appearance of a bone infection is a distinctive dark shadow; cavitation infections on the other hand give only a faint indication of their presence on an x-ray and are mostly overlooked. These infections can be painless or just the opposite, causing trigeminal neuralgia like pain. This pain is often mistaken for toothache and innocent teeth are extracted one after another in a vain attempt to stop the pain. Even worse, healthy teeth are root-treated causing more focal infections.

Smell is another way of detecting cavitation infections. When a cavitation is opened, either one of the two very characteristic smells appears. The most frequently encountered is the smell similar to stale smoke, like coming into a room the morning after a particularly good party. The other smell is a pungent sour smell often encountered if opening into a sinus. These smells are sometimes present when extracting teeth and when cleaning out periodontal or gum infections. The significance of these smells is not known, but they are another confirmation of the presence of a chronic long standing infection.

The most reliable way of finding out the size and position of a cavitation is without doubt the Cavitat Ultrasound Scanner. The Cavitat scan shows the true extent of a cavitation infection in 3D. It has revolutionised the diagnosis of cavitation infections and is probably the most important advance in dentistry in the last 20 years. The Cavitat takes the guess work out of cavitation surgery and increases the chance of a successful result.

THE CAUSES OF CAVITATION INFECTIONS

Cavitations occur when the blood supply is disrupted to bone. Injuries such as whiplash, falling of bikes or horses, are common causes of cavitation infections. Even falling into a taxi door 12 years earlier when drunk has produced cavitations in one of our patients. The blood supply can be interrupted by the trauma causing the bone to die which lets bacteria become established in the dead area. Dental injections, overenthusiastic orthodontic treatment, impacted teeth, infected or dead teeth and root fillings are other causes.

However, the commonest causes of cavitation infections are extractions. During extraction the local anaesthetic reduces the blood supply, the bone surrounding the tooth is fractured, and infection around the root surface is left behind. The socket closes and 'heals' leaving the bacteria behind to multiply and prosper. To protect themselves from the immune system, the bacteria wrap themselves in a slimy mucilaginous envelope. Here, they slowly expand like a balloon being inflated taking nutrients from their host and dumping their toxic waste products. The centre becomes hollow, hence a cavity is formed.

Such a process can take years; it is painless (usually), with none of the markers of an acute infection such as inflammation, redness, swelling, pain etc. Cavitation infections are seen in other bones after trauma and have long been recognised by orthopaedic surgeons. In children, cavitation infections are rare (the authors have never seen a case), probably due to the elastic nature of the young bone and the constant remodelling with growth. In young adults, 17+, they are quite often seen associated with impacted or un-erupted teeth. Diagnosis is by x-ray with experienced eyes or with an ultrasound scanner called a cavitat. Even pressing the fingers either side of the suspected area and eliciting pain with an increase of pressure shows the presence of a cavitation. By definition, a cavitation infection has a hollow centre, so the cavitat scanner can detect in 3D the size and position of a cavitation infection within the jaw bone.

Cavitations are more often found after wisdom teeth extraction and in back (molar) teeth extraction sites.

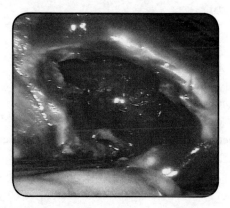

Fig. 3.15 A cavitation hole in the upper jaw. The gum has been peeled back and the soft bone scraped away. No drills were used to open the bone. The cavitation hole is approximately the size of a medium grape. The teeth were extracted 10 years previously.

The effect of these infections should not be underestimated as illustrated by the following three cases.

75

CASE STUDY 8

A young male, 21 years old, had all his wisdom teeth extracted at the age of 19 in hospital without undue complications. After a successful 18 months at university, he became chronically fatigued, was unable to concentrate, had an increase in allergies and had to stop studying. He came to us 18 months after ceasing to study in an effort to get his life back together. We had treated his mother successfully the previous year for a different complaint. Examination showed cavitations had formed around the sites of the wisdom tooth extraction; otherwise a sound dentition and no gum disease. The cavitations were opened and cleaned under the V-Tox protocol. Within a month there was a dramatic improvement in symptoms, and within six months he had resumed his studies eventually to graduate and start work. The symptoms completely resolved within 12 months, he got his degree and he lives a normal life.

CASE STUDY 9

The symptoms and causes

A middle-aged woman had chronic pain in her upper jaw for over 10 years. She went the rounds of all the relevant specialists and tests. No-one could find any reason for the debilitating pain. The only relief was the traditional treatment of antidepressants and tranquilisers which dulled but did not eliminate the pain. However, after 10 years, the side-effects of the drugs on the skin and digestive tracts were severe and increasing in severity.

The treatment and recovery

An examination revealed a large cavitation in the upper jaw where the pain was situated. Three teeth had been

76

extracted here several years before the onset of pain. The cavitations were opened and cleaned out using the V-Tox protocol. The upper jaw bone had rotted through into the maxillary sinus: the air space in the cheek bones. Within the space of a few weeks, the pain diminished and she withdrew on her own volition from all medication. After six months, the side-effects subsided, the pain disappeared, and she could get on with life again and has remained trouble-free to this day. Testing of the sample from the cavitation showed it to be extremely toxic.

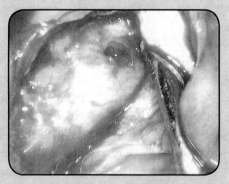

Fig. 3.16 The surface of the cavitation when the gum was peeled back.

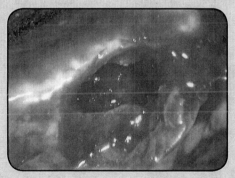

Fig. 3.17 The cavitation hole in the bone after the soft bone had been scraped away.

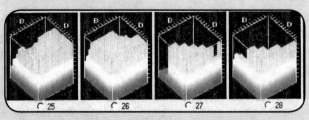

Fig. 3.18 A cavitat scan. Black denotes infected area; light grey is the bony borders of the cavitation.

CASE STUDY 10
The symptoms and causes

A female, 20 years of age had four wisdom teeth extracted at the age of 18 due to pain. There were no problems after the extractions. She had adult orthodontics for two years to straighten the upper teeth with a fixed railway track appliance. This was removed a year before we saw her. She had to give up studying due to chronic fatigue, inability to concentrate, stabbing acute pain in the jaw joint area, and around the wisdom teeth extraction sites that came and went. She had a sour taste constantly in the mouth ever since the wisdom teeth extractions that she found very difficult to bear. Many extensive tests had been performed but no diagnosis was made or help was ever offered. She had no fillings and no gum disease. The orthodontic treatment had given her pretty teeth, but the way the teeth fitted together was not in harmony with the jaw joints. A severe malocclusion, or structural stress in other words, was present. The jaw joints showed wear as they were forced back into the skull.

78

The treatment

The malocclusion we could fix first by a plastic appliance worn over the teeth, ending up with equilibration or grinding the fitting surfaces of the teeth to the correct shape.

A cavitat scan and OPG x-ray (a panoramic scanning dental *x-ray)* showed large cavitations around all the wisdom teeth extraction sites stretching under all the molar teeth. These cavitations were cleaned, but all were large and had spread to the neighbouring teeth.

The recovery

This cleaning only gave a minor relief. The patient wanted all the molar teeth to be extracted and the cavitations under them cleaned. We knew from the scan and the first operation that the cavitations involved the molar teeth, so these molar teeth, all unfilled, were extracted and the cavitations cleaned over a series of operations. Each operation brought more relief from the symptoms. After the final operation, leaving a 20-year-old girl with no molar teeth, her symptoms were resolved. No sour taste, no pain, no chronic fatigue etc. She resumed her studies and the symptoms have not returned. The missing teeth were replaced with partial dentures.

The trade-off between health and teeth

For her, the treatment was a success; the loss of the molar teeth was unfortunate, but better to have no molar teeth than no quality of life. These were *her words, not ours.*

There is no other way of treating such infections other than removing the teeth and cleaning the bone. The bacteria are entrenched and impervious to attack by either antibiotics or the immune system. Removing these teeth may seem a drastic step, but there was no other option. Conventional medicine had failed her; the infections shown on the cavitat scanner were real, and there is only one way of treating such infections. Essentially she made a trade-off: health for teeth; and in her case it worked out well.

The removal of seemingly healthy teeth without good justification in the hope of health improvement is never recommended. This is where experienced hands and proper testing are a vital requirement to good treatment.

Future treatment may be light pulse therapy as certain wavelengths of light can penetrate the slimy coat and kill the bacteria. However, this technology is not available at present, though the authors are conducting experiments with it. She was unfortunate to have bacteria in her cavitations that attacked the neighbouring bone so quickly. Possibly, the orthodontic treatment moved the teeth into the cavitations which speeded up the expansion process. Without a cavitat scanner it is doubtful we would have realised the true size and shape of the cavitation infections.

Out of interest, the extracted molar teeth were cut in half to examine the nerve or pulp inside. In the teeth next to the original wisdom teeth extractions, all the nerves had gone: the teeth were dead. In the next teeth along, all the nerves showed damage, none were healthy. Interestingly, all these teeth tested 'alive' on pulp testing before the extractions.

POTENTIAL SOLUTIONS TO CAVITATION INFECTIONS

Homeopathic nosodes

A popular approach to treating cavitation infections by some of the alternative dental community, but should be discouraged, is homeopathic nosode injection into the affected area. This just spreads the infection to deeper areas in the bone. There is no justification for such treatment. We have seen many cases of failed nosode injections performed by enthusiastic, but essentially ignorant practitioners. Homeopathic nosodes may be suitable in some situations; however, we do not use them. Our experience is that it is best not to pussyfoot about with bacteria, but go for them with all guns blazing.

Ozone

Injecting ozone into the cavitation reduces the bacteria numbers for a while, but because the bacteria are protected inside their slimy coat, the ozone cannot reach them all, so the infection returns as it was before, in a short period of time. It can offer short-term relief of symptoms, but it is not a magic bullet. Ozone is best used as one of the weapons to attack bacteria. Since the bacteria inside these cavitations are mainly anaerobic, oxygen is deadly to these bacteria and ozone is excellent in killing them if it can reach them. We use ozone as part of the treatment because it is so effective and the bacteria can never become resistant to ozone as they can towards antibiotics. Ozone is a significant part of the arsenal against bacteria, but using ozone injected into cavitation infections without other treatments will not work long-term.

Surgery

The inside surface of a cavitation is covered in a slime. This can be granular, sometimes discoloured and usually with very little, if any, bleeding.

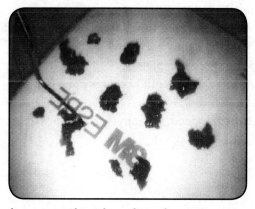

Fig. 3.19 The slime-covered inside surface of cavitations.

The bone surface is soft and has to be scraped away until healthy bone is reached. As some cavitations are larger than a thumb tip, this requires perseverance, time and a little courage on behalf of the surgeon to clean out thoroughly. Cavitations often follow nerve paths through the bone and it requires skilful handling not to damage a nerve and permanently lose feeling in the face. Cavitations can spread from one tooth area to involve neighbouring teeth.

The only way of dealing with these infections is surgery. Antibiotics will not penetrate the coating around the bacteria, neither will other agents such as ozone, gas etc. These antibacterial therapies can inhibit the bacteria but, in the author's rather extensive experience, never eliminate them. Surgical cleaning and washing have to be done. Washing with ozonated magnesium chloride in a 3% solution offers the best results. Bubbling ozone through the solution puts oxygen into the cavitation to kill the bacteria, and magnesium chloride rinse is a first world war tip to clean wounds. It disinfects and promotes the immune system in the area to speed healing. In some cases, when the immune system is compromised, other intervention is required.

2. Root fillings or root canal therapy

Root fillings are routine dental treatment. When the nerve or pulp inside the tooth becomes infected, it can die. Trauma or a blow to the tooth can cause the pulp to die as well if it disrupts the blood supply to the tooth.

Conventional wisdom says that
1. removing all the pulp tissue from inside the tooth,
2. sterilising the empty canal and,
3. filling the space completely,

can 'save' the tooth. The tooth becomes pain-free and the treatment is claimed as a success. However, the three objectives of root-filling are never fulfilled; indeed, it is physically impossible to do so.

82

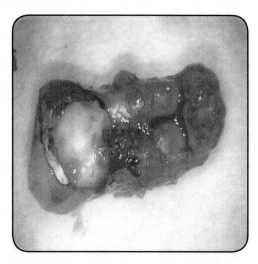

Fig. 3.20 A root-filled tooth showing build-up of bacteria in mucilaginous coating around the root tip and sides. This tooth was pain-free, but a major source of toxins.

THE INSIDE OF A DEAD TOOTH

The typical drawing of a tooth root shows a nerve inside the root joined to the main nerve under the tooth by a single strand. However, the inside of a tooth is not a single chamber; rather, the shape of the nerve or pulp is more like a plant root with lots of side shoots or lateral canals; or imagine a river delta, there is the main stream and lots of little streams all emptying into the sea, this is what the root tip is like. Plugging the main hole or stream will not plug all the little side streams or holes, it is impossible to remove all the nerve tissue from these side canals. Inside these lateral canals, the nerve tissue rots away, unable to be cleaned out. This rotting tissue becomes infected and no antibiotic or chemical can reach these bacteria. There is no blood supply, so the immune system cannot reach this area and the bacteria are allowed to live unhindered. Each root has more than 3km of smaller tubes that start from the nerve and end on the outside of the root. These tubes are microscopically small, but large enough to provide shelter for bacteria. Imagine cave dwellings long and thin where sunlight cannot penetrate and you will get the idea.

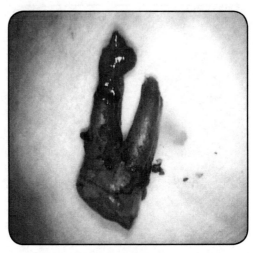

Fig. 3.21 An infected 'blob' of tissue on a typical root-filled tooth. Note the root-filling material poking through the root on the right.

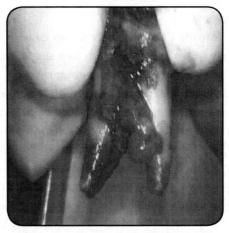

Fig. 3.22 No root filling could reach the infection between the roots of this tooth.

THE TOXICITY OF ANAEROBIC BACTERIA

Gangrene is the correct description of these infections. With no blood supply to any part of the former nerve, the bacteria that live there become anaerobic: this means they can live without oxygen; indeed, oxygen will kill them. These bacteria live and multiply. They produce waste which they dump. This waste consists of complex protein toxins. These toxins enter the body and can end up anywhere. The toxins from a root-filled tooth could be measured using a TOPAS test when this was available. This test collected fluid from around the neck of the tooth and analysed the degree of toxicity and the activity of the bacteria. This test is not freely available anymore. The complexity of the proteins is in proportion to their toxicity. The standard toxicity test uses mustard gas as a reference on a scale of 1 to 10 where mustard gas is 1. Frequently the toxicity of the bacterial protein is higher than 10 on the scale. Why have a piece of dead and rotting tissue just inches away from the brain? Where else in the body is dead tissue not cut away? If a finger tip died, would it be mummified, a new nail stuck in position, painted the correct colour and the patient told all was well? Certainly not!

Toxic root-filling materials

The trouble does not stop with the infections around the root-filled tooth. A variety of root-filling materials are used to fill in the space where the nerve was. As already explained on page 57, some are so toxic that it is forbidden to throw them away in case they contaminate water supplies. Other materials release formaldehyde and ammonia. Side-effects noted from root-filling materials are drowsiness, dermatitis, allergy, neurological symptoms, thyroid dysfunction, various pains, sinusitis and cancer to name just a few.

When a root-filled tooth develops an infection at the root tip or apex, an apicectomy is performed. This means cutting off the root tip and filling the space where the root tip was in the vain hope that this will remove the bacteria. In the UK, this is done with amalgam, but this is forbidden in Europe. This, of course, turns things from bad to worse. All apicectomies are infected, all are producers of toxins.

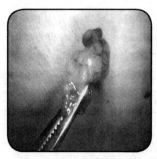

Fig. 3.23 Infected tissue removed from the bone where an apicectomy had been done.

'The location of the tooth, the types of organisms inside it and the nature of the person's genetic make up will determine the areas of disease found clinically. The one thing that is certain is that if you are sick you should look very carefully at all non-vital teeth, whether root therapied or not.'

Dr Gammal, Australian dentist and author of *Rooted*. See *www.rooted.tv*.

BIOLOGICAL ROOT FILLINGS

Biological root fillings consist of a calcium expanding paste of high pH. The paste will kill any bacteria on contact. It is placed into the pulp chamber and expands as it sets. This expansion forces the material through all the little tubules pushing the bacteria out. That is the theory. The bacteria are forcibly evicted from their caves to be killed by the immune system with the excess material being absorbed back into the body. However, theory and practice are not always good bed fellows. The material, Biocalex or Endocal, can only be used on new root fillings. A tooth cannot be re-root filled as the tubules will be blocked by the first attempt at a root filling so the Endocal will not be able to get into the tubes to evict the bacteria. Endocal cannot be seen on x-ray easily unless Yttrium is added to the paste. Proper filling of the canal is not done due to the complex shape of the pulp chamber. The authors experience is that, in the best of circumstances, one out of three teeth root-filled with Endocal, test toxin-free. The other two will remain highly toxic.

3. Extractions

The key to extractions without having a cavitation infection form afterwards is as follows:

- Extract the tooth as gently as possible: expand the bone rather than fracturing it.
- Remove by scraping as much of the infected tissue from the socket as possible, wash and clean the area.
- Try not to use a drill to clean out the bony socket, this puts micro cracks in the bone for bacteria to hide in.
- Use local anaesthetic without adrenaline to keep a good blood supply to the healing bone.
- Rinsing the extraction site with ozonated magnesium chloride solution.

It is an unfortunate fact that most adult extractions end up as cavitation infections to some degree. Some sources estimate as much as 90% of adult extractions end up in this way.

4. Gum disease

Periodontal or gum disease is an infection of the gum around the teeth. This starts in the soft tissue and eats away at the bone supporting the teeth until the teeth become loose and fall out or are taken out.

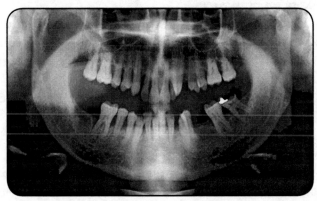

Fig. 3.24 A typical case of periodontal disease. Note how the bone has shrunk away from the necks of the teeth. This x-ray shows horizontal and vertical bone loss.

Periodontal disease is the commonest disease in humans affecting the majority of all adults and is the major reason for loosing teeth. It is a very serious infection and has been connected to strokes, heart attacks and even low-weight babies from mothers with periodontal disease. The DNA of the bacteria associated with periodontal disease has been found in the breakpoint of arteries in stroke victims even though the bacteria themselves were not found. Bacteria from the periodontal infections got into the blood stream and found their way to a place where the flow of blood was the slowest: on the bend of an artery. Think about fish in a river, they gather where the current is the slowest which is at a bend in a river. The current is faster one side of the river than the other side.

The same applies to bacteria in the blood stream. The bacteria set up a colony and the toxic release of the bacteria, remember heat shock protein 60, weakens the artery wall. At some point the wall will fail, and that is called a stroke. Research by Dr Vojdani showed the DNA of these bacteria to be identical to the DNA of mouth bacteria. Testing shows these bacteria to be extremely toxic. Amalgam encourages periodontal disease; more than that, it is one of the causative agents of periodontal disease. Periodontal disease is a known side effect of amalgam.

How Periodontal Disease Takes Hold

Periodontal disease starts with soft plaque accumulating around the necks of the teeth. This causes inflammation, or gingivitis, and the gums bleed when brushing. The gum around the teeth normally has a cuff (space) 2mm deep. This cuff deepens with the gingivitis creating a periodontal pocket which allows more plaque to build up creating more inflammation and so on. When the bacteria establish a colony and produce toxins, the body knows that this is a bad situation and responds by trying to isolate the bacteria by pulling away from the infection. It makes an enzyme that dissolves the bone from around the necks of the teeth in an effort to retreat from the source of the infection. Unfortunately, the infection keeps pace with the bone loss until all the bone is lost, the teeth become loose and eventually fall out. The original soft plaque is removable with good oral hygiene.

A reduced nutritional state, plus exposure to toxins (amalgam fillings for example) can predispose a patient to periodontal disease; so the answer is more than just good oral hygiene. But it is vital that you brush your teeth effectively as if your life depended on it because, in a broad sense, it does.

CALCULUS

The hard calculus or tartar that is scraped off by the dentist or hygienist is different altogether. These are deposits of calcium and mean that the underlying body chemistry is out of balance. If the pH of the body is more acidic than it should be, the key pH regulator mechanism removes calcium phosphate from the bones and uses the phosphate part to regulate the blood pH. The calcium part is a waste product and it is dumped; some of it around the necks of the teeth. The removal of calcium phosphate weakens the bones causing osteoporosis which is a disease of civilisation; it is not found in 'primitive' societies.

MEDICAL TREATMENT

Doctors give you drugs. It is what they are expected to do and they have little choice but to fulfil that role. No drug cures anything. The purpose of drugs is to relieve symptoms. A drug would not be a drug if it did not have some effect on the body. All are to some degree toxic and have to be detoxified in the liver. Drugs add to an overall toxic load, but they do have a place in treatment. It is sometimes as important to treat the symptom as to address the underlying cause.

Paracetemol, for instance, may stop a headache even if the underlying cause is a jaw joint dysfunction, (TMD). Correcting a jaw joint problem may take months so removing the headache with a drug is entirely appropriate. Paracetemol is toxic, especially to the liver. An overdose of paracetemol can irreparably damage the liver causing death. This is very sad in attempted suicides as the patient initially recovers from the overdose only to die a few days later from liver failure when perhaps the circumstances that had driven them to the suicide attempt were brought more into perspective and they no longer wanted to die. The side effect of drugs is an established fact and the number of drug related injuries and deaths from properly prescribed drugs are far higher than makes for comfortable reading. This is no diatribe against drugs, they have their place, but today's medical practice puts an over reliance on drugs rather than finding the root cause of the patient's condition.

Why allopathic medicine is dominant

The reason for this is partly the pharmaceutical industries' pursuance of profit, which is why they are in business, where sometimes profit is put before ethics. Another reason is the public's demand for a quick fix or immediate gratification. The public expect to receive a prescription when visiting the GP, and usually do so; they also are conditioned by pharmaceutical media hype to think that that drugs actually work in curing diseases. It is partly the doctor's fault for allowing themselves to be seduced by the pharmaceutical industry, giving in to economic pressure from their various paymasters and to the expectations of their patients. Drugs are more part of the problem than part of the answer.

Challenging the status quo

How did it get like this?

> 'Most men can seldom accept even the simplest and most obvious truth if it would oblige them to admit the falsity of conclusions which they have delighted in explaining to colleagues, have proudly taught to others, and have woven thread by thread into the fabric of their lives.'
>
> Tolstoy

What must not be true, cannot be true. This is the attitude of organised dentistry. How can organised dentistry admit that the cornerstone of its treatment, amalgam fillings, is dangerous to health? How can they admit to focal infection theory when it will open a huge can of worms with regard to root fillings and cavitation infections? It is difficult to step out of the party line as the penalties for doing so can be draconian, such as a career cut short. Also, medical and dental egos are developed to such a degree that to challenge a long held belief is seen as a personal attack on the doctors and dentists and the institutions they represent.

Just look what happened to Dr Wakefield when, far from challenging vaccines, he suggested that they should be looked at in the light of emerging scientific data in relation to gut inflammation and autism. He did not say that vaccination was dangerous, nor that it should be stopped; he just wanted a rigorous scientific investigation of the facts. He was ruthlessly and continually professionally attacked, accused of professional misconduct at the GMC and had to resign from his job. He had committed heresy by challenging the current view on vaccines and vaccination and heretics must be punished to put fear into others who may want to challenge the status quo. Vaccination is a religious dogma of medicine as fluoridation is a religious dogma for dentistry. Speak up against it at your peril.

There is a lot of group fear in the mental make up of academics and those in authority and it is an unwritten imperative not to rock the boat. It becomes self perpetuating because those who do not subscribe to the view of the herd soon find themselves isolated and outside the group. These individuals are invariably found in general practice outside institutions. The established dogmas of treatment take on a religious aspect. They cannot be challenged as that is heresy. Fluoride is a perfect example of this in the dental profession. The science showing that fluoride is harmful, especially to ethnic minorities, is overwhelming. The science that shows fluoride is effective in reducing tooth decay is doubtful in the extreme, and that is being kind to it. Even so, the dental profession, initially against fluoride, supports water fluoridation with a zeal that is so contrary to the facts that it has become an article of religion, not science. What brave soul in academia would dare stand up against this and still expect to have a career?

Cherry-picking data

There is also a great tendency to cherry-pick scientific results to support a particular opinion. By this we mean an opinion on a subject is upheld by only looking at reports (no matter how dubious) that

91

support it and ignoring any reports to the contrary. One would hope and expect that all the science is examined and judgements made after examination of all the facts, but plainly this does not happen. It always takes time for new ideas to be accepted; there is always a deal of inertia to overcome beforehand, but sometimes inertia leads to active obstructionism. This is true in all human endeavours of course, not just medicine or dentistry, but medicine and dentistry pay lip service to science and we think they are being dishonest to the public. The amalgam controversy is a perfect illustration of this.

Standard of care

Standard of care is another vehicle of attack; I know, it has been used against me – (G M-H). Standard of care was originally used to protect practitioners who may not be on the cutting edge. How it worked was like this: If a new piece of science was reported in the literature that a practitioner did not know about, he could not be attacked by a smart lawyer saying that this science was published last month, yet you did treatment xyz to my client which is contrary to the published science. The practitioner could say that in the profession overall, treatment xyz was the norm. If you went to 100 practitioners, 99 would do as he did, e.g. treatment xyz, whereas only one practitioner would follow the new science. Therefore treatment xyz was the standard of care.

When used as a weapon of attack, the standard of care is turned on its head. In this instance, the practitioner who used the scientific evidence and could prove the validity of what he did, can be accused of malpractice because if a patient went to 100 practitioners, 99 would do the old treatment and only one would use the new scientific method. Therefore, the 99 must be right and the one must be wrong even if the evidence supports the one. Sometimes, we are sure this world is just a big Mad Hatter's Tea Party and we are all having tea poured over our heads. As an aside, the hatters were mad because they suffered from mercury poisoning. The term quack treatment was to describe those who used quicksilver or mercury in treatment. This too has been turned on its head. I (G M-H) was accused of quack treatment by a consultant neurologist because I suggested that mercury released

92

from amalgam fillings that was above the European limit may have a neurological effect on a patient. Question: Is mercury the most neuro-toxic naturally occurring metal on the planet? No prizes for getting that one right. There is a lot of tea being wasted poured over people's heads.

SUMMARY

- There are many toxic materials used in dentistry.
- Amalgam is the worst as it emits mercury vapour into the body.
- All materials have a potential for harm, but dental alloys contain heavy and transitional metals which are especially reactive to the body.
- Implants are usually metals, though non-metal zirconium implants are gaining in popularity. Bacteria can migrate into the space between the implant parts and allow chronic infection to establish itself.
- Poor dental function, as well as inadequate nutrition, compounds the problem by lowering the tolerance to any health disturbance.
- Focal infections can cause symptoms in the body far away from the site of the infection.
- Cavitations, root fillings and extractions are the prime sources of bacteria, i.e. focal infection. These bacteria are isolated from any attack
- Gum disease is very prevalent in the adult population and is a major source of toxin releasing bacteria.
- Dental metals and bacterial toxins can have devastating health consequences.
- The condition caused by the toxins is not predictable due to the complexity of the toxins and the genetic makeup of the patient.
- Medical treatment can only treat the symptoms not the cause of the problems created by toxic dental materials.

4 THE SOLUTION

This section will outline the procedures for the patient. It is not a definitive fully-complete explanation. It will give the patient a good idea of what to expect and why. It will also give a practitioner a glimpse of what the public will come to expect, hopefully, in the not-too-distant future.

The procedures are described in a little detail so that the potential patient has enough background to question a practitioner and assess whether the practitioner is capable of delivering safe effective treatment. Practitioners, dentists or medical doctors who want more detail will be able to find it in an upcoming book: *A Manual of Holistic Dentistry*. There are no secrets that we are holding back, anything we have learned in the crucible of experience is to be freely available to any who seek it.

WHAT IS TRUE HOLISTIC DENTISTRY?

The term 'holistic' is sadly much abused. Part of the solution is the application of holistic dentistry as we understand and practise it. Being a holistic dentist is not, as one of our patients once said of other practitioners he had been to, putting a crystal in the window and calling themselves holistic!

Holistic dentistry:
- is an integration of conventional and alternative therapies to promote optimal health as well as to prevent and treat disease;

* includes all safe and appropriate modalities of diagnosis and treatment;
* includes the analysis of physical, nutritional, environmental, emotional, lifestyle components of the patient;
* uses patient education and participation in the healing process;
* will search for the underlying causes of disease rather than treating symptoms alone.

Holistic dentists:
* expend as much effort in knowing the patient as they do in finding out what kind of symptoms the patient displays;
* will influence patients by their own example;
* view illness as a manifestation of a dysfunction of the whole person and their past, not as an isolated event;
* will show the way to release the emotional toxic consequences such as hostility, shame, greed, depression, fear, anger, grief and lack of self-love;
* are lifelong students.

Simple holistic dentists are passive. They:
* do not use toxic materials in treatment;
* do not use treatment methods that harm the patient (or are the least harmful);
* carry out a full examination, know their patient, come to a diagnosis and make a treatment plan appropriate to them.

Complex holistic dentists are active as well as passive. They:
* remove toxic material safely from the teeth and jaws;
* remove and treat all infections safely;
* repair the damage wrought by toxins on the patient.

V-TOX THERAPY

V-Tox describes treatment protocols that can be justly described as complex holistic dentistry. V-Tox was named by a German lady who worked for us who said one day, 'You have to call this baby something. You use vitamins and you detoxify patients so why not call it V-Tox?' Since no-one else had any better suggestions, the name has stuck. V-Tox was developed over the years to treat the ultra sensitive and complex patients in a safe and effective way.

Safe and effective treatments were necessary because we saw patients treated by well-meaning practitioners ending up in hospital after having amalgam removed. We have witnessed neurological symptoms flare up and one poor soul even ended up in a coma for 30 days after repeated DMPS injections (to remove mercury from the body) from his 'holistic' dentist; not by us we hasten to add.

So it became rapidly apparent that removing the toxins without damaging the patient required very careful planning and preparation. The dental part needed a practitioner to be highly skilled with considerable experience, and a lot of adjunctive therapies were needed. All the treatments we have developed are based on science and applied using our extensive experience. It took some time before all the elements necessary for success were understood and for us to fully comprehended the complex nature of the therapy we had developed. We can proudly say most of the patients improved, but no-one became worse after the treatment.

In brief, the therapy is as follows.
- Examine the patient.
- Do the appropriate tests.
- Make a treatment plan based on the results of the above.
- Know what the end result you want is, both dentally and generally.
- Work out the order of treatment and the materials used.
- Prepare the patient nutritionally.
- Use intravenous vitamin C and glutathione at high doses during all the treatment.
- Do all invasive dental work over a two-day time period if possible.
- Remove all metals from the teeth.

- Make sure the teeth, jaw joints and jaw muscles are working in harmony.
- Eliminate infections.
- Use special dental treatment protective protocols, e.g. oxygen, when removing metals and treating infections.
- Aftercare: make sure the gut is working properly.
- Any other sensible treatments that may be required are prescribed, e.g. cranial osteopathy, colonic irrigation etc.
- Follow up at three, eight and 18 month intervals at least. Have some yardstick to measure progress, e.g. symptoms, tests, pH, questionnaires etc.

Homeopathy, acupuncture and all other similar therapies are best done after the patients have had their toxins removed. The various therapies may help, but nothing will hold or permanently help the chronically ill patient until the patient has removed the malign influence of the toxins from the body. All these adjunctive therapies have far more success when applied *after* the V-Tox therapy rather than *before* it. Otherwise it is a bit like pushing water uphill, a lot of effort and not much to show for it.

Examining the patient

It all starts with information gathering. The forms the patient fills in beforehand give the practitioner an idea of what he is facing (note: all the forms we use are available on the website *www.toxicdentistryexposed.com*). Gaps in information are filled in by questioning the patient at the examination appointment. This examination process takes some considerable time, anything between one and three hours including any tests that need to be done. What the practitioner needs to know is what the main problem the patient has and what the patient wants and expects. The level of patient awareness, attitude and therefore compliance is critical. Certain patterns do appear. Patients with mainly a mercury problem will differ from patients with a substantive infective problem, for instance.

This will be a story for another book, but it needs to be established if the main symptoms are from:

- infection (tooth, bone or gum);
- toxins, i.e. poisoning;
- sensitivity (allergy);

or a mixture of them all.

Doing the appropriate tests

Having understood the background and nature of both the condition and the patient, certain tests may be needed. A word of warning here: Testing a sick patient will give the results of a sick patient.

What this means is that a test may show the effect of the toxins on the body's biochemistry. Removing the toxins should bring back more normal readings. Test results can indicate the nature of the problem being faced, but no treatment should be started based on test results alone. Do not start treatment to bring back normal test results before removing the cause of the poor test results, i.e. toxic load.

Generally, it is better to test a patient *after* treatment to see what needs to be done in order to obtain optimum health. This is opposite to modern medical practice which bases treatment on test results, but this 'test and prescribe' mode of treatment is better suited to symptom relief rather than getting to the heart of the problem; the toxic load of the patient. Tests are also a significant income source for the practitioner.

Take pH, for instance. If the pH levels are too high, the wrong way round, or too low, it would be a mistake to start a course of treatment to alter the pH until the toxins have been removed. The pH levels only indicate that there is an underlying problem. Treat the problem, not the symptoms. Remove the toxins and most of the time the pH will regulate itself.

If after treatment there is still a pH irregularity, that is the time to begin specific pH treatment. This will appear contrary to modern thinking of testing, diagnosing on the test results and prescribing the drug of choice, which is what most us have experienced in modern medical practice.

THE PATIENT IS ALWAYS RIGHT!

At least 50% of patients come with a dossier of test results all of which are 'normal', but they are still sick. Worse off are the patients whose test results have improved with a particular treatment, but still feel sick. The doctors look at the test results, declare the case a success and dismiss the patient. If the patient protests at this, they are told one of the two famous medical phrases, 'It's all in your head' or 'Nonsense, you must be better now'.

No-one asks the patient these days in a meaningful way which is a great pity because at some level, depending on the background and awareness of the patient, the patient always knows what is wrong. It is annoying for the practitioner, myself (G M-H) included, who have to deal with their own ego issues, but *the patient is always right*.

THE TESTS

Some of the following tests may be necessary. The aim is to do the minimum of testing which is truly required; this limits the expense only. Before undergoing a test, patients should consider if the results will alter treatment in any way. For example, all amalgam gives off mercury and mercury always damages the body to one degree or another. The only point in having a mercury level test is to decide whether the levels are high enough to warrant having the amalgams removed or just for curiosity's sake. But what levels of mercury are 'high' for an individual patient? No-one knows the answer to that question.

Since there is no test that will show the individuals tolerance level to mercury as a poison, any test results are by and large irrelevant. Testing for mercury *after* amalgam removal, to see how much is still retained in the body, would be a better idea.

Cavitat scanner

The Cavitat scanner is an ultrasound device approved by the FDA. It can detect cavitation infections in jaw bones. The accuracy of the device is stunning.

Mercury level tests
BREATH

This is easily done at the chair side with instant reliable results. Several devices are available to do this. It demonstrates mercury release to the patient and gives a good indication of the degree of exposure to mercury from amalgam fillings. There are methods of calculating the body burden of mercury using a breath test.

STOOL OR FAECES

This is not popular in the UK, but it gives an accurate level of the body burden of mercury. Only specialised laboratories can do this. The level of any metal can be tested for.

SWEAT

A sweat test is difficult to do outside specialist laboratories, but is a good indicator of the body burden of mercury.

BLOOD

Useless; a waste of money, time and effort. It isn't accurate at all. Anyone who suggests a blood test is obviously ignorant about mercury chemistry.

URINE

This is about as useful as a blood test since the kidneys' filter mechanism distorts the actual level of mercury excreted.

KELMER (CHALLENGE TEST)

Here, the levels before and after the administration of DMSA (dimercaptosuccinic acid) or DMPS (dimercaptopropane sulfonate) are taken. DMSA and DMPS both release mercury by chelation and the amount released gives an indication of body burden. Such tests can be extremely dangerous for sensitive patients as they produce a lot of free mercury to flow around the body. Added to which, the kidneys are not designed for mercury excretion and can be damaged when mercury is forced through them. *This is definitely not a recommended test as many patients have been harmed using DMSA and DMPS.*

100

HAIR

A hair test is a good indicator of long-term exposure to all sorts of things, mercury included. However, the test must be done at a laboratory that does not wash the hair before testing as the hair is open to other topical toxins from the air (which are washed off) and shampoos etc. This means some caution needs to be used when reading the results. Furthermore, some individuals cannot detoxify mercury at all, so their hair analysis is misleading in the extreme; mercury does not appear in their hair, ever. This is especially seen on autistic children whose body tissues are loaded with mercury, but none appears in their hair analysis. The real problem is their lack of detoxification ability, not low mercury levels.

Sensitivity tests

SKIN PATCH TESTS

These are useless to the point of actually being dangerous. We have seen many patients made ill by such testing. The degree of accuracy is about as good as tossing a coin; *definitely not recommended.*

LTT (LYMPHOCYTE TRANSFORMATION TEST)

It tries to correlate reactions of the lymphocytes (white blood cells) to various toxins, mercury included. It has been superseded by the far superior MELISA test.

MELISA TEST

This is a blood test that can very accurately measure the sensitivity or allergy type response to a host of different metals and pollutants. If considering any metal dentistry, this test should be done to establish any reactions to the metals proposed to be used. It is useful to establish proof of allergy or sensitivity if that is required. Always bear in mind that if you have not been exposed to a metal before, the test may say this metal is safe for you, but over the years, sensitivity to this metal could build up. Repeated testing is recommended if you are a metal wearer. Scientifically the MELISA test is the *gold standard* of blood tests.

Take a small piece of the material in question and place it in the mouth between the cheek and the teeth. Start with five minute durations and build up to 30 minutes. Take a one hour break between each test. Observe any reactions that may take place such as local irritation or a generalised symptom such as tachycardia (accelerated heart beat). This is a crude, but generally reliable test to see whether an individual can tolerate any particular material. Especially useful when testing for cement compatibility.

APPLIED KINESIOLOGY (AK OR MUSCLE TESTING)

This can give a good indication, but depends on several variable factors such as the experience of the practitioner. Only use as an indication, do not count on its reliability.

EAV (ELECTRO ACUPUNCTURE ACCORDING TO VOLL) OR ELECTRO-DERMAL TESTING

This involves interpreting skin voltage fluctuations when a substance is put into a circuit with the patient. Generally, EAV is not that convincing. We have sent the same patient to different EAV practitioners and got a different result every time. However, we do know of one practitioner whose results always agree with other test results we do. She has proven to be extremely reliable, so there must be something in it, but it is a minefield. How do you know if the results are reliable or not from any particular practitioner or machine they are using? You pay your money and take your choice on this one.

Other tests

ALT BIOSCIENCE

This laboratory used to test for bacterial toxicity using biopsy samples from cavitations, root-filled teeth and even the fluid around the gingival cuff. The test measured the degree of inhibition of six energy enzyme systems in the body. The higher the degree of inhibition of the enzymes, the greater the toxicity present. This was a measure of toxins released from bacteria and was very reliable and accurate. Hopefully, similar tests will be available soon. (See *Fig. 3.13*, page 69 for typical results.)

NEUROPATHY PROFILE

This is a blood test from BIOLAB, London. It measures different minerals and enzyme systems. Different neurological conditions show specific profiles. This test is useful in measuring progress and for nutritional targeting of specific minerals and amino acids. (See page 129 for more info.)

PAGE BODY BIOCHEMISTRY

It measures blood calcium and phosphorus levels. Only use fasting results. It shows the degree of biochemical imbalance and chronic inflammation present. It is a very useful monitoring tool, but only available from very few practitioners now.

PAGE BODY MEASUREMENTS

This is a another test to assess underlying hormonal predisposition. This is stunningly accurate, but obtaining the hormonal correctors in the dilution required has proven to be difficult. It is certainly a test to fine tune health after toxin removal.

BLOOD BIOCHEMISTRY

It is good as a snapshot of general condition. ESR (erythrocyte sedimentation rate) is a good indicator of chronic inflammation for example. Raised liver enzyme levels are a red flag; this means trouble is brewing.

pH

The blood pH needs to be stable at 7.34. If the blood is below this, it is called acidic; though chemically speaking, it is alkaline if the level is above 7. Blood pH is critical and can be measured, but it is tricky as several readings are required over many days to see a trend. The blood is taken, spun down and the pH of the plasma is read. It is easier to take the pH of urine and saliva. The patient can do this at home. It must be always done at the same time of day; morning and evening are best, but nothing must be eaten or drunk two hours before the test. Early morning levels are always more acidic than levels taken at 11.00 o'clock which is the optimum time for taking

103

a reading. The levels should be 6.5 to 7 for saliva and 0.2 lower for urine. Mild fluctuations are normal and depend on the diet of the day before. Wild fluctuations of over 0.5 are not good. Even worse is a urine pH level consistently higher than saliva pH level. This shows a chronic disturbance in the body, usually of many years, and indicates, in our experience, a deep seated viral infection. A significant minority of such patients will require other treatment to tackle such deep seated intruders.

METABOLIC TYPING

This establishes your individual metabolic type. Different types require different foods to keep optimum pH levels in the body. Literally, one man's meat is another man's poison. This takes just over two hours to do and must be done while fasting. A measured amount of a type of glucose (or protein) is drunk, and over the next two hours, changes such as blood sugar, respiration, saliva and urine pH, pulse rate, blood pressure etc. are measured. There are three basic metabolic types; each type requires different foods to maintain a stable pH, and therefore, good health.

These types are as follows.
- Protein type (type 2) – the typical North European type who requires animal protein (non-muscle protein is especially good) at every meal time. This type does badly on grains, sugars, certain vegetables, exotic fruits and processed foods.
- Carbohydrate type (type 1) – virtually the opposite of the protein type in simple terms. This type does well on grains and most vegetables.
- Mixed type (type 3) – the lucky ones; they are a mixture of both types and provided that they don't overindulge in any one food group, they can eat most things.

A metabolic typing test shows whether a patient:
- is oxidative or parasympathetic dominant;
- has a fast or slow metabolism;
- is acidic or alkaline;

104

- is dehydrated;
- has catabolic or anabolic cellular processes.

It also shows aspects of cell membrane regulation (and other technical stuff). The best time for this test is after treatment, not before. The metabolic typing test is recommended for assessing changes in the diet to achieve long-term good health.

FAT BIOPSY

Fat is taken and analysed for pesticides, herbicides, fire retardants and other chemicals associated with modern life. If the levels are regarded as high, phospholipid therapy along with intravenous vitamin C and glutathione is indicated. This is quite a long-term therapy, but is effective in reducing the levels of chemicals absorbed in the body; the lipid or fat soluble ones, at any rate.

GENETIC

A genetic test can show a predisposition for certain conditions. Alzheimer's is a good example. Having a predisposition does not mean that contracting the disease is inevitable. The test does give a patient time to develop a prevention strategy against certain conditions.

CANCER

There are a number of tests available, not recognised by regular oncologists, which give an indication of approaching cancer. They also serve to show if a particular therapy is working or not. Some are blood tests while others are urine.

THYROID

A thyroid test is a blood test for thyroid hormones or thyroid antigen. Individual variation will mean that, for some patients, a low but normal level is in fact too low for the hormones. Basal temperature taken first thing is a good indicator of thyroid health. If it is low, something may need to be done. Do not mess with the thyroid, get expert evaluation. There is controversy between the American test for triiodothyronine (T3) and the Europeans' test for thyroxine (T4) to measure thyroid efficiency. The American approach is the more logical one of the two. Temporary tweaks of the thyroid are possible during treatment especially as mercury is a thyroid inhibitor, as is fluoride.

Quite often after V-Tox treatment the thyroid function improves dramatically. This is due to the removal of mercury bound to the thyroid which is inhibiting thyroid function. If selenium is deficient in the diet, and it usually is, mercury will attach to the thyroid where selenium should be. If sufficient selenium is taken, the mercury will be dislodged by the selenium as the thyroid, given a choice between mercury and selenium, will always choose selenium. Thyroid antigen tests detect whether the body is destroying the thyroid itself, for example Hashimoto's Thyroiditis. This has been successfully treated by V-Tox therapy.

LIVER FUNCTION

It can be useful as it indicates which of the four major phase II detoxification pathways is not functioning properly. There are nutritional ways to enhance each individual pathway. A major use of the test is to find out the ratio between phase I and phase II detoxification pathways. Phase I takes toxins in the body and makes them water soluble and ready for the phase II pathways to finish the job of detoxification. If phase I is elevated and phase II depressed, the bioavailability of the toxins is enhanced. This greatly increases the danger to the patient. If the position is reversed and phase I is depressed, then phase II pathways cannot function properly anyway.

MISCELLANEOUS

This includes measuring antioxidant status, glutathione peroxidase levels, red cell mineral levels, and gut porosity.

A WORD OF CAUTION

Individual variation means that what would be normal for one patient is abnormal for another. All results have to be read bearing this in mind. Just because the result is within a normal range does not mean it applies to all patients. The normal range is highly suspect too as it is derived from establishing a mean set of results from blood tests done in hospital. After all, that is where most of the blood tests are done. However, the blood tests in hospitals are done on a range of patients who are already sick, otherwise they would not be in hospital. So normal levels are really an average of the results of sick people and may not apply to everyone.

If the test results are improving, but the patient is not feeling or seeing the improvement, it is time to re-evaluate the treatment strategy because something significant may have been missed. It could be psychological such as the patient forgetting how bad they were in the beginning or they need the illness as a control mechanism over family and friends and will never feel better. It could be physical such as a chronic gut dysbiosis (microbial imbalances) that has been overlooked or a cavitation infection is still present. This is where the experience of the practitioner plays a major role.

Hard tissue evaluation

After gathering all the information from tests, the hard tissues are evaluated first. These are teeth, bones, jaw joints and sinuses. The teeth are examined for metals, levels of occlusal (bite) stress, wear pattern and function to each other and to the jaw joints. Root-filled and dead teeth are noted. It may be necessary to take models of the teeth and mount them on an articulator to have a working representation of the mouth. Any alterations planned can be practised beforehand on the model and any problems noted and a solution found. This is an excellent diagnostic tool.

The jaw bones are examined for signs of infection and periodontal (gum) disease. Infection may be seen at the tips or apices of the teeth, in between the roots of molar (back) teeth, on extraction sites and in cavitations.

Jaw joints are examined for wear, noise on movement, irregular movement and disc wear or displacement. A judgement has to be made whether changes seen are irreversible or reversible. If reversible, decisions must be made on how this can be reversed and if irreversible changes are present, how comfort and function can be best achieved.

The sinus spaces in the upper jaw, are looked at to see if they are cloudy which may mean infection or have the tips of the teeth sticking into them. Chronic sinus problems will have been picked up earlier on in the examination, so this can be confirmed. Conventional sinus treatment, lavages, stripping etc., is a waste of time and highly uncomfortable as well. The way to healthy sinuses is to establish proper drainage. There are a variety of ways available for this. If the teeth poke through into the sinus space, infection in the sinus may cause symptoms in the tooth. X-rays will be necessary.

Usually, a panoramic x-ray is taken and maybe individual films as well, in order to show all the teeth. Digital x-rays give an immediate picture and use much less radiation. However, the quality of the digital image is only now coming close to the quality of a well-taken and processed conventional film. CAT scans and 3D imaging use a lot of radiation and their use in the everyday situation is limited. The problem with CAT scans and 3D imaging is that if metal is still present in the mouth, it causes radiation scatter which can lead to misinterpretation of the results. These types of imaging are best done in a metal-free mouth.

A WORD OF CAUTION

Practitioners see what they are trained to see and what they want to see. If a practitioner does not believe cavitations exist, he will not see them. This is true of panoramic x-rays, CAT scans and the like. Often overlooked is condensing osteitis around the root tip of a tooth. A typical infection at a root tip shows up on an x-ray as dark space; this is the everyday apical infection. In a chronic or long-term infective situation, the bone has grown thicker around the root tip: it has condensed. This is more of a danger to health than the dark apical infection and trickier to spot as well.

Dr Hans Nieper, a German cancer specialist, believed that condensing osteitis was connected to the onset of cancer. Whether this is true or not we, the authors, do not know. However, all the adult cancer patients we have seen have had condensing osteitis or cavitation infections in the mouth. The reverse does not hold true: not every condensing osteitis or cavitation infection patient gets cancer.

Obviously there must be other predisposing factors and time needed before a cancer starts.

Cavitation infections can be seen on panoramic x-ray films, but not always. Sometimes the film may only hint of a cavitation infection and not be definitive. This is the time to use the cavitat ultrasound scanner. This device, in experienced hands, gives an accurate 3D image showing the size and location of the cavitation infection. Our experience with a cavitat scanner is that if it shows a cavitation on the scan, there is always a cavitation present. Occasionally, it will not show a cavitation that is present, but this is more likely due to operator error or peculiar local conditions than any fault with the cavitat itself.

Digital thermography which detects heat output is a new promising technology that may prove to be useful in screening for dentally related infections. The jury is still out on the long-term usefulness of thermography but it most probably will turn out to be a good indicator of dental infections.

Soft tissue evaluation

Soft tissue evaluation involves assessing the gums for gingivitis or periodontal disease, measuring periodontal pockets, gum bleeding, tooth looseness etc. Chronic infections are checked for and any metallic tattoos noticed. A gum tattoo is a dark mark on the gum; these are called amalgam tattoos in common parlance. Occasionally, they are in fact due to pieces of amalgam stuck in the gum when an amalgam filling breaks during an extraction. This is, however, quite rare.

A tattoo is really a concentration of metal ions. An infection produces an electrical charge locally in the gum and this attracts oppositely-charged metal ions. As the amount of metal ions increases, the tattoo becomes larger and darker, very often seen around the incision marks of an apicectomy (where the tip of a tooth root has been cut away).

Tattoos need to be surgically removed, no matter how large they are or their position in the mouth. All are prime evidence of toxic load. This can be quite a task as the tattoo is usually infiltrated with stringy connective tissue and around the edges are lots of small round dark areas of tissue. All the dark matter must be removed. With large tattoos, this can take a series of operations to remove it all. The largest tattoo we have removed covered over a third of the lower jaw and went down to the bone. Removing the tattoo gave a fast and significant improvement of health. We had to remove it as the patient's local dental hospital refused to operate due to the size of the tattoo and we knew that unless it was removed, the patient could not possibly recover. All tattoos are signs of active pathology and should be removed if at all feasible.

Treatment planning

Using all the information gathered, a treatment plan can be worked out. This will include a precise idea of the dental result and the overall desired health improvement. The dental result means what will happen to each tooth and the overall function of the teeth and jaws within the physiological limits of the patient. The general health picture relates to the specific needs of the patient, which must be identified beforehand. Reference points must be built in to measure progress or lack of it. Without reference points of some sort, it is difficult to accurately gauge the effectiveness of the treatment. After recovery begins, patients easily forget the state they were in when they first attended. This is where photographs and symptom charts prove to be invaluable.

Such symptom charts are subjective, and careful judgement is called for. For instance, we had an MS patient many years ago who claimed that there was no difference to his symptoms after treatment. About three months after treatment at a recall visit, he left the practice and walked 1km to his parked car. He then came back to the practice because he had forgotten his support walking sticks at the practice. He was shocked when he realised what he had done as this showed him how much he had improved over the time. As the improvement was not dramatic, he had not noticed the gradual improvement in stamina and balance. In such a case, a good reference point would be distance walked without support. Each case has to be taken on its own merits.

The order of treatment should be written down, i.e. gums and jaw joint first, then teeth, and then the surgical removal of infections would be a typical case. Each patient will be different. Any adjunctive or additional therapies such as ozone or cranial work or gut dysbiosis or other therapies will also be factored in. This is not a simple task and can be quite daunting to a professional starting out in this field. The next step to consider is the appropriate materials to be used for the teeth and perform any testing that may be indicated.

Treatment protocols

Only now can any actual treatment commence. Patients are somewhat shocked and annoyed when they ring our practice and try to book an appointment for amalgam or metal removal and we say 'No'. We need to see and get to know the patient first to find out what needs to be done and whether we are the right ones to do it. It is also important to find out if the patient is ready for us as well.

By this we mean that the patient understands what we are doing and why we are doing it. Occasionally, someone will ask for one part of the treatment, but not want another part of the treatment. This indicates that they either do not understand the concept of what we are doing or think they are a 'special' case for one reason or another. This pick from a menu approach never gives the best result for the patient.

AMALGAM AND METAL REMOVAL PROTOCOLS

IAOMT (International Academy of Oral Medicine and Toxicology) has established the recommended minimum treatment protocol for the safe removal of dental amalgam. These should be used whenever amalgams (or other dental metals) are being removed. The point of these protocols is to minimise the amount of mercury released and absorbed by both the patient and staff when drilling out an old amalgam filling. These protocols are the following.

- The patient breathes a separate air or oxygen supply.
- The operator and staff wear mercury absorbing masks.
- The patient wears eye protection.
- Amalgams are 'chunked out', not grounded out.
- High speed drills are used with copious amounts of water irrigants and coolant.
- The air in the operating room is filtered to remove mercury vapour.

111

- Rubber dam or 'clean up' tips are used to isolate the teeth during amalgam removal.
- The patient's skin and clothing is covered, with minimum skin area exposed.
- The mouth is constantly rinsed to remove amalgam particles and mercury vapour.
- High speed suction in use in the mouth at all times.

Failure to observe these rudimentary steps will increase the mercury exposure of a patient. Naturally it goes without saying that the debris collected, old amalgam etc. must be responsibly disposed of to protect the environment. The regulations about waste mercury are quite stringent because it is recognised by the various environmental agencies as an extremely hazardous substance. In fact, the only safe place to store or use amalgam is in the mouth; *Alice's Adventures in Wonderland* made real!

THE V-TOX PROTOCOLS

The V-Tox method uses the IAOMT protocols, but goes further.

1. The patient must be prepared using appropriate supplements.
2. Intravenous vitamin C with glutathione is always administered to the patient during or immediately after metal or amalgam removal for one to four days afterwards. The amount of vitamin C will depend on the weight and condition of the patient, but a minimum of 0.75g/kilo body weight diluted in Ringers Lactate and 800mg to 1500mg glutathione is used in every infusion. In some cases two infusions are given daily.
3. Any form of surgery will require special measures against bacteria, such as ozone, magnesium chloride rinses, etc. The reason we do all these extra measures is because of the dramatic effect they have on the patient. Healing is quicker, often the pain is less and the dangers of infection all but eliminated. Vitamin C and glutathione bind and remove mercury successfully and safely from the body.

The preparation phase

This will vary a little from patient to patient but the basic principles are described here. The pH and basal temperature is measured for a week beforehand. This will be repeated three months after treatment and compared as a measure of progress. The patient receives one of two basic packages of supplements. One is VTP3 powder with oils. The other is MP oil and powder. The list of ingredients of VTP3 is on *www.toxicdentistryexposed.com*.

After treatment, the supplements continue for another month. We prefer that patients stay on this supplementation for at least three months but eight months is better. Some patients keep taking it forever. The aim of supplementation is to increase antioxidant levels, regulate pH, and promote proper gut function. If the gut is not working and regular, eliminating the toxins is nigh on impossible. Diet recommendations are given as well. These are to eliminate sugar and refined flour completely. Take butter and yoghurt but reduce or eliminate milk, increase the number of eggs and good protein. No alcohol (that is a form of sugar), no caffeine and no undiluted fruit juices. Drink clean mineral water, a minimum of one litre a day.

Mercury is very reactive to the phase I detoxification pathway, and phase I can be elevated using alcohol. This is why, in the authors view, dentists working with mercury have always had a tendency for high alcohol consumption. Drinking helps the dentists remove mercury from their bodies and they feel better. Every working day they expose themselves to mercury by placing and removing amalgams without sufficient protection, so they have a constant need for alcohol.

Keep on this diet during the preparation and treatment phase and stick mainly to it afterwards as well. Metabolic typing after the treatment will refine the correct diet to follow for life. Following this preparation protocol has increased our success rate substantially as well as helping patients have a healthier life afterwards.

Sugar addiction is surprisingly high and many have to be weaned off sugar with Stevia. Stevia is a South American herb that can substitute for sugar and has positive health benefits. Chocolate is always mentioned, especially from the choco-addicts. If whole organic chocolate is taken in moderation, even the raw variety provided no sugar

113

or milk is added, chocolate can have health benefits. Eaten this way it is impossible to binge out on chocolate.

Cavitations

Cavitation infections or NICO (Neuralgia Inducing Cavitational Osteitis) lesions are holes in the bone caused by anaerobic bacteria. The bacteria produce toxins which are dumped into the body. The bacteria arise from infected teeth or infected sites after a tooth has been extracted. The only truly effective treatment for such infections is to open them up and thoroughly clean them. Injecting ozone into a cavitation can temporarily limit toxin production as ozone kills many of the anaerobic bacteria contained within the cavitation, but the walls of the cavitation are covered in a gelatinous slime made by the bacteria to isolate themselves from the body's immune system. The ozone cannot penetrate through the slime to reach all the bacteria. Some survive, and when the ozone is used up, which it quickly is, the bacteria are back in business. It is only a matter of time before things are as they were.

Extractions

Extractions are a major cause of cavitations. Cavitations occur when infected material is left behind in a tooth socket. An infected tooth often has a 'blob' of infection hanging under the root tip.

CASE STUDY 11

The size of some of these cavitations is quite frightening sometimes. The first one we ever cleaned went from the first premolar tooth to the wisdom tooth area in the lower jaw. About one third of the jaw was hollow. Very occasionally dramatic results happen when a cavitation is opened. On this occasion the lady patient in question, who had insisted on the operation despite our misgivings (before the Cavitat was available), suddenly sat upright and shouted, 'That's it, you've got it!' as soon as we had opened her cavitation and exposed the contents to air.

She frightened the life out of us at the time, suddenly sitting up and shouting, but her symptoms of chronic fatigue and multiple chemical sensitivity began to diminish almost immediately. We knew the size of the cavitation from a CAT scan, but the picture did not do justice to what we actually found.

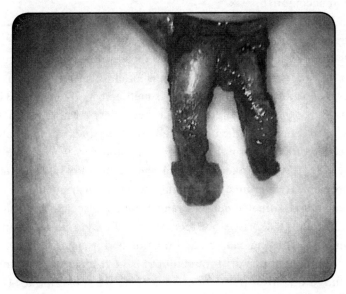

Fig. 4.1 A typical infected tooth with a 'blob' of infection hanging under the root tip.

If a tooth is extracted and this infected 'blob' remains behind in the socket, the blood clots in the socket sealing the infection in place. The bacteria organise themselves and a cavitation infection starts. If part of the membrane that holds a tooth in place is infected and left behind, that too can form a cavitation. If the bone surrounding the tooth is cracked or traumatised during the extraction, even of a healthy tooth, that will reduce the blood supply to the bone. A reduced blood supply and trauma to the bone are the classic ways of forming a cavitation.

THE V-TOX METHOD OF EXTRACTING A TOOTH

Statistics are hard to come by, but Cavitat Medical Technologies, Inc. report that around 80% of all adult extractions end up as cavitation infections. This figure we would support from our own experience. The figure is higher for wisdom teeth extractions. The V-Tox method of extraction tries to be as gentle as possible, neither leaving infected material behind nor cracking the bone. It does take some considerable time to accomplish.

In brief, the membrane holding the tooth in the bone is cut or separated. A series of hand instruments gently widen the bone around the tooth. The tooth is then rocked to increase the widening, but all the time very gently. The final stage is either levering the tooth free with an elevator or with forceps. This method usually keeps the blob on the end of the tooth. If the blob has been there a while, it will have grown and eaten away the bone around the root tip creating a hole up to the size of a finger tip. In this case, the blob may tear off and stay in the hole. It is important to try and remove the blob intact so as not to spread bacteria around the wound site. Hand instruments are used to clean out all infected debris in and around the socket. Drilling the bone to remove debris is not recommended unless no other option is available. Drilling can spread infection and traumatise bone. The school of thought that drills out 2mm of bone from around the socket to remove infection in the bone is not one we subscribe to. Drilling always produces fractures in the bone. Cracks in the bone are a perfect hiding and breeding place for bacteria and cause cavitation infections later on.

After careful extraction and using hand instruments to remove infective debris, the socket is then washed with a 3 to 5% magnesium chloride solution that is ozonated. Ozone is bubbled through the solution to sterilize and saturate it. Repeated rinsing kills the anaerobic bacteria lining the walls of the cavitation. Anaerobic bacteria live without oxygen, exposure to oxygen will kill them. A solution saturated in ozone is an effective way of dealing with dental infections. The magnesium chloride has other benefits too, by itself it is an antiseptic but it also stimulates the immune system locally which encourages trouble-free healing. This is an adaptation of Dr Pierre Delbet's treatment of wounds initially developed in the First World War.

The socket is then filled with a base layer of ozone gel. This gel acts as a bactericide but is quite runny. On top of this gel, a thicker gel of antibiotic paste is applied. Blood infiltrates and clots in the mix and the socket is sewn over. We have the various gels made for us by compounding pharmacists (those who make their own medicine). Using this technique we have eliminated most of the problems associated with extractions and later cavitation formation. Very little swelling or after pain occurs using this extraction technique, but it does take some considerable time and care to perform. DMSO, a solvent, can be used in combination with antibiotics as it is a pain reducer in its own right, but has drawbacks too. The gels have to be freshly mixed for each patient.

EXTRACTING WISDOM TEETH FROM THE UPPER JAW

Upper wisdom teeth extractions are notorious at forming cavitations. The bone around these teeth is called the tuberosity; it is not as densely compacted as the bone in the lower jaw, and a cavitation infection very often renders the tuberosity to be completely hollow.

When extracting the tooth immediately in front of the empty wisdom tooth site, the second maxillary molar, as the elevator is levering the tooth backwards, quite often the tooth will fold into the bone or tuberosity behind it. The tuberosity is hollow and the extracted tooth has collapsed backwards into the space of the cavitation. Infection spreading forwards from the wisdom tooth cavitation can infect the second maxillary molar which is why it needs extraction. When such an event happens, the dentist, if he cares to look, sees that the bone has rotted to such a degree that he is staring at what appears to be the base of the skull. That gets the dentist's heart racing along nicely!

More information on ozone

Ozone has many uses in holistic dentistry. It kills bacteria and supplies oxygen to tissues. It is made up of three atoms of oxygen.

117

The oxygen gas that we know and breathe is made up of two atoms of oxygen, which is stable; three atoms are not stable. Ozone is highly reactive and breaks down to oxygen. When it does this, it becomes an oxidising agent and this is how it destroys the bacteria. It can deal with MRSA, the hospital superbug, and no bacteria can ever become resistant to ozone, unlike chemical antibiotics and disinfectants. It can be used as a disinfectant to wipe surfaces, to kill bacteria in cavitations, periodontal pockets and extraction sockets; and to stop decay on teeth and disinfect root canals. It is not expensive either nor is it patentable. Since little money can be made with ozone gel it is little known and used.

Ozone as a Gas

It is useful as a gas, a gel and as a saturated solution, but breathing ozone gas is not recommended as it produces severe coughing fits and will damage the lungs. The gas has to be used with care to make sure the patient does not inhale it. That said, many ozone practitioners do inhale very dilute concentrations of ozone gas themselves claiming health benefits from this, but we suggest this is not a wise thing to do.

Ozone Administered Intravenously

Ozone can be used intravenously as well. The action is similar to intravenous hydrogen peroxide in that both decompose to produce oxygen (hydrogen peroxide producing water as well). Intravenously, the objective is to increase the oxygen supply to the body in order to increase metabolic efficiency, reverse any anaerobic metabolism as seen in cancer cells, and to kill any stray organisms it finds. Intravenous ozone will increase the immune system efficiency if given at the correct dosage, but it can, if given for too long at too high a concentration, reduce the efficient working of the immune system. Ozone gas can be injected into a vein directly, popular as a self-administered therapy in AIDS patients, or blood is taken out of the body, ozone bubbled through it and the blood put back. The Russians and Cubans use saline or Ringer's solution instead of blood to bubble the ozone

118

through and inject it back into the body. Major and minor autohaemo-therapy is the name for the two ways of administering ozone.

Ozone is a controversial topic in medicine, mainly because there is no patent on it which means no-one can make money from its manufacture. If safe ozone practice was freely available in the medical system, the health benefits would be absolutely enormous to the public at large. Nearly as much benefit to the world at large as intravenous vitamin C, which is our next topic.

Intravenous vitamin C

Intravenous vitamin C is the cornerstone of V-Tox therapy.

> 'There is nothing intravenous vitamin C cannot cure if given long enough and in high enough doses.'
>
> Dr Frederick Klenner, the pioneer in using intravenous vitamin C

Our experience over the years has proved Dr Klenner to be, by and large, correct. Intravenous vitamin C really is that good. Intravenous vitamin C and ozone cancel each other out. Ozone is an oxidising agent and vitamin C is a reducing agent. They cannot be used together at the same time. Ozone grabs electrons whilst vitamin C donates them.

This is not the place to go into the chemistry of vitamin C; what it does and how to use it are more important to the reader. Vitamin C is essential for life. Scurvy is the disease of vitamin C deficiency. The scourge of sailors in the past, scurvy was responsible for tens of thousands of deaths. To stop scurvy, a very small amount of vitamin C is needed, around 65mg per day is the recommended level (RDA).

VITAMIN C AS A HEALING AGENT

For maintenance of health, far higher doses are required: at least 1000mg a day. On a personal note, the author has used vitamin C daily for close to 30 years at a dose of 10,0000mg (10g) to 20,0000mg (20g) a day to remove mercury and recover from his heart condition with only positive effects. Vitamin C is wholly positive, it accelerates healing.

119

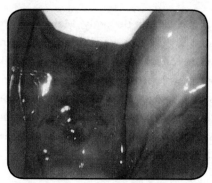

Fig. 4.2 Operation site 24 hours after cavitation operation. Note the accelerated healing response due to intravenous vitamin C.

Those who say otherwise are scientists who use dirty glass in their experiments as happened at one UK university, or the pharmaceutical industry who rightly fear reduced sales of drugs if people took more vitamin C.

Vitamin C, or ascorbic acid, to give it its proper name, is acidic and can upset digestion causing pain and some degree of flatulence due to its acidity. This can be overcome using magnesium ascorbate or calcium ascorbate instead. 20% more of these ascorbates will be needed to have the same effect as pure vitamin C.

How it works

Vitamin C is a reducing agent; it removes metals from the body not by chelation, like DMPS, DMSA or EDTA, but by oxidation/reduction reactions similar to what the body does. Chelation, on the other hand, chemically grabs the metals and minerals, and strips them from the body including all the essential minerals such as magnesium, copper etc. This is the danger of chelating agents, especially long-term use or one should say abuse.

Two comments about chelating agents: The manufacturer of DMPS say that DMPS should be used for acute mercury poisoning only, not chronic exposure to mercury as comes from amalgam fillings. DMPS should be used twice in two weeks then not again for six months because of the dangers of mineral depletion. This sound advice is ignored by many practitioners.

EDTA is too weak to remove mercury, it has not got enough chemical energy to break the mercury bond which is a tenacious one. EDTA as a mercury chelator is ineffective. Vitamin C works by donating an electron. This is essentially what anti-oxidants do. Mercury when it is bound to tissues is forced to accept an electron from vitamin C and when it does, it loosens the bond and becomes free. Imagine a mercury atom hanging on by one hand like a monkey to a branch in a tree. Along comes vitamin C and gives the monkey a banana (an electron), the monkey grabs the banana but then falls out of the tree. Mercury in this state is not so reactive and will find it difficult to rebind to tissues. While it is in this state, glutathione wraps the mercury securely up and takes it to the colon where it is excreted.

Now for the really clever bit. After glutathione does this, it needs regenerating to be able to wrap up more mercury. Regenerating glutathione requires an electron from vitamin C. So if there is enough vitamin C available, glutathione keeps on regenerating and removing mercury and a host of other toxins as well. A virtuous circle is created. This is why V-Tox protocol adds glutathione to the intravenous vitamin C infusion to super-charge the detoxification of mercury and other toxins from the body.

Vitamin C also re-hydrates cells making them go back to their proper shape. Cells function properly only when they are the correct shape because they interact with the body messenger hormones by a lock and key mechanism on the cell membrane. This is simplifying things a little to make it readily understandable. Not only this, but vitamin C powers up the mitochondria which are the energy suppliers of the cells. This allows the cells to work at a high rate of efficiency. Allied to vitamin C's power to kill viral and bacterial infections, all this makes vitamin C a powerful weapon in the arsenal to obtain and maintain optimum health.

ORAL VITAMIN C DOSAGE

Vitamin C given orally can cause looseness of the bowels. This is called bowel tolerance, which will vary from individual to individual and the degree of ill-health of that individual. For example, the author came back from holiday in Sri Lanka. There he had made friends with Michael, the hotel's python. However, on the flight back, the author came down with a severe fever of rapid onset, probably caught from Michael. Back home, he took 120g of vitamin C over 24 hours before any looseness occurred in the bowels. The next 24 hours this was reduced to 70g vitamin C before looseness occurred, and the third day he was back to 30g. The fever had completely dissipated by the third day. The progress of the path back to health could be measured by the amount of vitamin C taken. The more ill the patient is, the more vitamin C is required before bowel tolerance is reached. This is a somewhat uncomfortable way of using vitamin C, but none the less effective for all that.

INTRAVENOUS VITAMIN C DOSAGE

Vitamin C used intravenously has an entirely different effect. Intravenous vitamin C or IV-C, actually sucks water out of the bowel and, instead of producing looseness of the bowel, has a tendency for constipation. However, this is mitigated by the thirst patients generate when undergoing IV-C. This thirst must be satisfied with good quality water. There is a threshold value for the amount of intravenous vitamin C needed for therapeutic effect. This fact is not well understood by the medical profession, a lot of whom think 1 or 2g of intravenous vitamin C is sufficient. This is the standard dose for treating burn victims, but it is wholly inadequate. 100g to 200g daily would have a much greater beneficial effect.

The threshold dose is 0.75g vitamin C per kilo of body weight. This is the minimum; under severe toxic conditions this can go up to 1g per kilo of body weight. In patients with severe cavitation or other infections, we will give two intravenous vitamin C infusions at this high dosage on the same day. This speeds up the rate of healing enormously, reduces the risk of infection, reduces the chance of post operative swelling, bruising, and reduces pain. The highest amount of intravenous vitamin C we have ever given is 250g a day for three days. It was given to a Gulf War victim suffering from Gulf War Syndrome for just over a year. This was at the patient's request. He said he felt good with a normal IV-C but 'knew' his body needed more.

At the end of day three he said, 'That's enough' and his symptoms had gone. A word of caution here, Gulf War Syndrome is many faceted, and what helps one, may not have the same effect on another. Also, treating him shortly after the war was to his advantage rather than after many years of suffering, which would reduce the patient's recovery potential.

As was already stated, we use it diluted in Ringer's lactate solution. One part vitamin C to four parts Ringer's is the dilution ratio. The vitamin C for intravenous use is buffered to make the pH compatible with blood. Saline can be used instead of Ringers, but it is not as good. Using saline as a diluting agent can cause dizziness and a feeling of disorientation in some patients. Ringer's lactate mimics plasma and the electrolytes are in the same ratio as found in the blood which gets over this problem. The infusion is given at a rate of 72 drops a minute; this means an average infusion will last between two to three hours.

WHEN NOT TO USE INTRAVENOUS VITAMIN C

The only contra-indication to intravenous vitamin C is G6PD deficiency. G6PD is a liver enzyme but it is rare to find deficiency. We have come across it only twice in over 20 years. It is found usually, but not always, in persons of Eastern Mediterranean or African descent. G6PD deficiency is mostly picked up after severe reactions to antibiotics. This is not to be confused with allergy responses to antibiotics, which are fairly common. A simple blood test can check to see if G6PD deficiency exists. It is not usually tested for unless there are good reasons for doing so. If a patient goes to the GP and receives an antibiotic, the doctor does not check for G6PD beforehand and the reactions, which are severe, are the same for antibiotics as for intravenous vitamin C.

Kidney disease or dysfunction is often stated to be a contraindication to intravenous vitamin C. This is not the case; in fact, just the exact opposite is true. Initially, we did not treat patients with kidney disorders because we had read about the contraindication to vitamin C. However, patients became aware of this and would lie about their kidney condition in order to receive the treatment. We began to receive appreciative letters from kidney specialists noting the improvement in their patients after our treatment. Now we would recommend intravenous vitamin C for patients with kidney dysfunctions.

'SIDE-EFFECTS'

Patients always feel thirsty when having an infusion of vitamin C, and the first infusion is rather special. Patient's faces go very pale; the paler they go, the more toxic they are. This is a good sign, as it means the toxins are being released from the body.

'California cool' is the mental state of patients after the first infusion. It is called California cool because their anxiety has now gone; they are in a relaxed frame of mind and no longer uptight. During the infusion week, we have the saying, 'Come in like a lion, leave like a lamb' to describe the changes in attitude we see on patients during this week. Initially, patients can be angry, fearful, aggressive, and anxious. By day four, most of this has dissipated.

Practitioners with no experience of intravenous vitamin C often advise patients not to go through this treatment because they are not strong enough to withstand it. *This is always a mistake.* Intravenous vitamin C will support even the delicately balanced and seriously-ill patient throughout all the trauma of the treatment week. Patients should remember that without this treatment their chances of regaining their health are markedly reduced. As was stated before, we are quite often the 'end of the road' where patients end up when all else has failed.

THE USES OF INTRAVENOUS VITAMIN C

Dr Klenner used 7.5g vitamin C injections as his first aid tool. Whenever an unconscious patient was brought to him, he injected the 7.5g, as usually this brought the patient round to answer questions or bought him time to run lab tests to see what treatment needed to be done. We have used this method ourselves and can vouch for the effectiveness of it.

Intravenous vitamin C has been used successfully in treating the following ailments for many years.

- Drug overdose
- Snake bite

- Viral infections
- Bacterial infections
- Poisoning
- Auto-immune conditions
- Neurological conditions

We have added the following diseases to the above list using the V-Tox protocol.
- Acne
- Multiple chemical sensitivity
- Chronic fatigue
- Fibromyalgia
- Arthritis
- Allergies
- Psoriasis
- Ankylosing spondylitis

The list goes even further than this, but we don't have enough space to mention them all. The only one on the above list we have not had personal experience with is snake bite, but that is rare in Bedfordshire!

Why children die of meningitis is a mystery to us, especially as Dr Klenner's protocol is freely available and worked well for him in severe viral infections in children. Why not use it now to save lives at risk? It is easy to administer, inexpensive and effective when used correctly. The virtues of intravenous vitamin C are too numerous to mention other than briefly touch upon the subject here. More information is available on the website *www.toxicdentistryexposed.com.*

Why intravenous vitamin C is not widespread

If it so wonderful, why is not used more? The answer, as ever, is to follow the money. With no patent available for vitamin C, there is no financial incentive for any pharmaceutical company to make it or promote its use. Just the opposite in fact, as the use of vitamin C on a wide scale would damage drug sales and pursuit of the bottom line is the primary goal of any company or corporation.

Despite the books and articles written on vitamin C over the years, only a handful of practitioners use it. Medicine since the 1950s has always been anti-nutrition and pro-drug for a variety of reasons; so to advocate a vitamin for any reason has been to swim against the tide of prevailing 'expert' opinion and invoke the wrath of authority. This has changed recently as the American Dermatological Association has actually recommended vitamin D. Sunlight is slowly coming back into medical fashion after being demonised for many years. Helios therapy or sunlight was in medical vogue in the early-to-middle 20th century, before the skin cancer scare was foisted upon us. More people probably got a worse form of cancer from using the sunblock creams than they would have ever contracted from sunlight.

A cautionary tale

Once at a medical conference, we all had our antioxidant levels measured. Our antioxidant levels were four to five times higher than everyone else apart from the doctors engaged in cancer research. Their levels were even higher than ours. When taken aside and asked in private why this was, one doctor said, 'Because we know'. That was all he said. When asked why not everyone else could know as well, the answer was a chilling, 'The time is not ready yet'. No further comment from us is necessary, save to say how many must suffer before the time is right? How many lives will have been lost before the time is right?

SUMMARY

- Examine the patient properly.
- Write a treatment plan to remove dental metals and infections.
- Supplements are used to raise antioxidant status and regulate pH.
- Dental treatment is carried out over two days.
- Intravenous vitamin C is used at high doses and is administered for three to four days including the days of dental treatment. More infusions may be required.

- Keep a high level of antioxidants and minerals in the body for eight months.
- Monitor progress at three, eight and 18 month intervals.
- Additional therapies may be indicated.

THE SOLUTION IN PRACTICE

This chapter illustrates actual patient treatments. These are not theoretical discussions, but are just a few of the many cases we have been privileged to help over many years. This is not an armchair warrior scenario, but real cases with real results.

The starting point is with actual diagnostic descriptions such as neurological problems and allergies and so on. The treatment and outcome of patients with these conditions will be described in detail. Those who have persevered from the beginning of the book will realise that the distinction between conditions such as neurological, autoimmune, allergy etc. is, by and large, illusory.

The underlying cause of these MCDs is toxic overload and the label put on the display of symptoms the patient displays has little affect on the eventual outcome. The label can effect the patient's perception of their condition for good or ill and it is a handy administrative tool. It creates career pathways for medical professionals and is useful in planning and financial considerations. However, this does not alter the underlying fact that the label describing any MCD is an illusion.

Some of the cases illustrated will fit into several categories, while others will not fit into any category at all. Where a patient fits several categories, they will be mentioned in each category and a reference will be made to where the complete description of the case is. For instance, a neurological case may also be a chronic fatigue case, as well as a cavitation infection case. A detailed description will be available in the neurological section and the case will be referred to in the chronic fatigue section. In this way readers who are concentrat-

128

ing on any particular condition will be able to read in detail about the particular cases they are interested in.

V-TOX AND MODERN CHRONIC DISEASES
Neurological

The typical neurological cases we see are motor neurone disease (MND), Alzheimer's, Parkinson's, neuropathies (muscle weakness), and multiple sclerosis (MS). The major concern with these conditions is that by the time the symptoms are noticed and a label is given to them, so much time has passed that many of the patients are past the point of recovery. That is not to say that a significant easing of symptoms and reduction in the speed of progression of the diseases cannot be achieved in some cases.

MOTOR NEURONE DISEASE (MND)

Fat biopsies typically show MND patients to have very high levels of Lindane (a pesticide) and flame retardants from furniture and clothing. MND-like conditions have lower levels of these chemicals, but are significantly higher in organophosphates. If circumstances allow, phospholipids therapy may be indicated to reduce these levels; which would start after the V-Tox detoxification regimes had begun.

Biolab's Neuropathy Profile blood test shows different patterns of nutrient deficiency in different conditions. For instance, all neurological patients are short in gamma-tocopherol, but not in alpha-tocopherol; and nearly all are deficient in omega 3 and omega 9 essential fatty acids. Some MS patients are low in omega 6, but not the 3. Vitamins B1 and B3 are virtually always at a low level and so is B6 in half of the patients. Interestingly enough, folic acid and B12 are within the normal ranges, but need to be supplemented anyway as we find that it helps. Glutathione and its complexes are deficient in most patients, but mineral levels such as magnesium and zinc show no discernable pattern. The supplement regime designed for these patients must be adapted to address any nutritional deficiencies shown by the test.

A careful examination is required to identify the toxic areas and a plan is made for the removal of these areas. This will consist of removing all mercury amalgam and other dental metals. Infected teeth and bone must be removed and structural stresses alleviated. Long-term therapies such as the Klenner's protocol and Low Dose Naltrexone (LDN) must be considered after the initial treatment phase is over.

There are cases reported in the literature of recovery from MND after amalgam filling removal. It has to be stated that in MND, by the time treatment starts, it is usually too late to affect the eventual outcome.

ALZHEIMER'S

This disease is again time dependant, but early toxin removal followed by repeated intravenous vitamin C and supplements of acetyl-L-carnitine, lithium aspartate and lithium orotate would be our recommendation along with the antioxidant OSR, developed by Prof Boyd Haley. The Mercury-Alzheimer's connection is scientifically strong.

PARKINSON'S

The symptoms only become apparent after over 70% of the particular brain cells have become affected. High levels of mercury are found in the cerebrospinal fluid (CSF) because mercury damages the blood brain barrier allowing large complex molecules to enter the brain which otherwise would have been kept out; agro-chemicals to be specific.

Once again early interception seems to offer the best hope. Full recovery is doubtful, but significant symptom relief has been seen after aggressive detoxification and with the supplementation of OSR.

MULTIPLE SCLEROSIS

This disease can also be included in the 'Auto-Immune' section, but is generally classified as a neurological condition. Our experience with MS goes back over 20 years. Typically a young patient would come along with a diagnosis of MS and x-rays showing lesions in the brain. After treatment, new x-rays show the lesions reducing in size, along with the symptoms fading away, so the neurologists call it a mistaken diagnosis, because no-one recovers from MS.

130

The earlier treatment starts, the better the chance of recovery. Young patients with symptoms for less than seven years respond the best. Someone who is wheelchair bound for 20 years is unlikely to have the same healing potential left. However, that is not to say such a person can not derive benefit from treatment. One of the key factors is the mental strength and steely determination of the patient; without an abundance of these, little progress can be expected.

Some patients need their illness to use as a form of control and will never respond to any treatment permanently; other patients are beyond the point of recovery. Trying to identify either of these is tricky in the extreme. Once again, the key is identifying and removing the toxins correctly following the V-Tox protocol. This can be reinforced using Klenner's protocol and LDN.

Klenner's protocol was developed by Dr Frederick Klenner for MS, but helps with other conditions as well, especially myasthenia gravis where the effect is dramatic and rapid. Dr Klenner is the father of intravenous vitamin C therapy and was persecuted for his knowledge and perseverance by his colleagues. Briefly, the protocol consists of a specific regime of high-dose B vitamins and minerals taken orally along with intramuscular injections of liver extract, the latter twice weekly or every other day. The patient follows the regime at home, self-injecting. The regime is followed for as long as is necessary.

Low dose naltrexone (LDN) is a relative newcomer. This is taken by capsule in the evenings at doses between 3 and 4.5mg. With LDN, the patient is on the drug forever. Stopping taking the medication allows the symptoms to return. LDN works in a variety of ways, one of them being the stimulation of the immune system. The normal therapeutic dose for alcoholics and drug addiction is a 100mg capsule. At low dose, the effect of LDN is remarkably different. Sometimes no treatment will work, on other occasions the case can be quite simple.

Normally, for MS and similar patients, we try the simple approach first and only add the other protocols if we are not successful. Both Klenner's protocol and LND have to be funded by the patient or the patient's family; this continuing financial obligation can present a problem for some families.

CASE STUDY 12

The symptoms and causes

A young man in his early twenties came to us walking with difficulty and he was occasionally forced to use a wheelchair. The onset had been rapid over the previous two years with just a few periods of remission. He was an identical twin, his sibling had no symptoms. The summer prior to the onset of his symptoms he had worked in a heavy industrial plant and had been exposed to a mixture of aerosol pollutants. Added to this, his studies involved contact with complex hydrocarbons such as glues, acrylics, paints, solder etc. His sibling had never been exposed to these pollutants. Both of them had had mercury amalgam fillings for many years.

The treatment

We checked his pH of urine and saliva to work out his supplement regime. The amalgam fillings were removed and he had five consecutive high dose vitamin C infusions. He continued on the supplements afterwards for eight months.

The recovery

He was back at his studies within a few months as his symptoms slid away from him. He wrote to us telling us that the only thing that reminded him of his condition was a slight drag in the right foot, but he could run half marathons without difficulty.

He had youth, optimism and an early intervention on his side. He did not need any continuing protocols such as Klenner's protocol or LDN that other patients might need. It was the combination of mercury from his amalgam fillings, plus the industrial toxic exposure, plus the exposure to toxins at his studies that had combined to give him his

132

symptoms. His sibling, genetically identical, had amalgam fillings but no symptoms, because he had not had the same exposure to toxins as our patient had.

Case study 13

The symptoms and causes

This case is different and dramatic and shows that even the amalgam-free patients can have neurological problems. The patient was a high-flying business lady in her early 30s. She had a developed a tremor most noticeable in her legs but also in the arms and hands over the previous three years which had forced her to give up work. She also complained of poor skin with frequent infective eruptions. She had undergone every test known to medical science and ended up with the neurological diagnosis of essential tremor: a tremor that no-one knows the cause of. No treatment, conventional or alternative, had helped her at all.

She had no history of amalgam fillings, but did have two root-filled teeth as well as two metal (palladium alloy) ceramic crowns. The way the crowns had been made gave her structural stress as well. The root treatments had been done a year before the symptoms started and the crowns were placed a few months before the root treatments. The wisdom teeth were present and healthy, for once.

The treatment

All we did was the normal individualised supplementation: four vitamin C infusions when we removed the root-filled teeth and cleaned out the infected bone around the extracted teeth. A specialised bite appliance was made to immediately remove the structural stress. The metal in the crowns was a palladium alloy which we replaced with crowns made from Zirconium.

The recovery

Within a month, the tremors had stopped and she was back at work. It was likely to be the toxins from the bacteria around the root-filled teeth along with the palladium alloy crowns and the locked in bite in addition to a stressful, nutritionally poor lifestyle that had combined to knock her down. Her skin problems disappeared as well. We quite often see that palladium and mercury removal can restore skin to health. Palladium exposure seems to be the main culprit in skin problems as well as frequently causing thinning hair, especially on females approaching and beyond the menopause.

Altogether a dramatic result from a minimum intervention; she had spent far more money in consultations and tests with specialists than we charged her. She had no other avenue open to her apart from us which puts a great deal of responsibility onto our shoulders. Her comment was, 'Why don't people (i.e. medical and dental professionals) know about this?' This is an excellent question for which we have no answer; in Lilian's words, 'It is just housewives' common sense'.

Allergies – multiple chemical sensitivity (MCS)

Patients come to us after developing allergies over several years. These allergies become more serious and more numerous over time. Foods and chemicals such as personal care products like deodorants are the main offenders. The probable cause of this tidal wave of allergies we are experiencing in the developed world is the ever increasing and continuing exposure to chemicals of all descriptions. This exposure overwhelms the body's capability of dealing with the toxins, so allergies begin as a warning to stop further exposure. The allergies can

134

be open and dramatic like rashes, headaches, gut problems, mucous formation and the like; or hidden. Hidden allergies may not be immediately apparent, but cause long-term chronic inflammation. When the capacity to react to the allergies is overwhelmed, this sets the stage for cancer. We do not see many cancer patients with allergies, their immune system is too bankrupt to react to the allergens any more.

Identifying the allergens, wheat and dairy being the most common culprits, and avoiding them is the first step. Exposure to mercury lowers the immune system and the threshold to allergies. Children and babies inherit their mother's gut bacteria, allergies and, unfortunately, their toxins as well. In utero, the infant preferentially absorbs mercury from the mother, and as mercury from amalgam is concentrated in breast milk, the infant has a high exposure to mercury. The newly-born have an immune system that is not fully developed. Faulty gut bacteria and a high toxic load can easily overwhelm the fledgling immune system. This is a cause of infantile dermatitis. This is as distressing to the parent as it obviously is to the infant. These cases came to our attention when we were treating a parent who raised the question of what to do about their child, who was not responding quickly enough, if at all, to the conventional creams and potions. Lilian has devised a special infant supplement powder which, when given in conjunction with our live gut bacteria culture grown on an oatmeal base, rapidly eliminates the problem.

Lilian too, suffered multiple allergies that grew extreme over time. The removal of an infected tooth resolved her problems, whereas auto-vaccines made her problems worse. Auto-vaccines may be all well and good, but the basic rule of allergy treatment is to stop being exposed to the cause of the allergy rather than attempting to become desensitised to the cause. There are many examples we could have given involving mercury amalgam fillings alone, but we wanted to show that mercury is not the only offender in causing these types of problems.

CASE STUDY 14

The symptoms and causes

A young woman in her late twenties had a weeping, itchy rash over large parts of her body. The rash started about six years before and had slowly grown larger and more unbearable. A constant round of steroid treatments helped keep things in check, but that was all. She had several metal-bonded crowns, but no cavitations or root-filled teeth. Interestingly enough, the crowns were placed two years before the rash developed. She had over time also developed multiple sensitivities to most foods. She had experienced an auto-vaccine treatment at a specialised clinic which had made the problem worse.

The treatment

There was no way of knowing what metals were in the teeth until we took the metals out. Rather than perform a series of expensive tests to check for metal allergies, we decided to take the metals out. Testing for allergies on such a patient with a hyped-up immune response would not have given accurate results anyway as she would react positively to almost everything. We replaced the metal crowns with crowns made from a glass and ceramic mixture. This is non-reactive to the immune system, but does emphasise hot and cold temperature transfer into the teeth. Like other cases, she had individualised supplementation and five days of consecutive vitamin C infusions as we replaced the metals.

The recovery

The rashes faded away within six months as did a lot of the other sensitivities. They faded in waves; by this we mean they reduced, came back a little but never as strongly, and then faded even more. This was a repeating pattern

136

and we have seen it with a lot of patients. We analysed the metal in the crowns and found out they were made using a silver/palladium alloy. Subsequent testing showed her to have a sensitivity to palladium.

This case was our introduction to the kindling response. The kindling response describes what happens to a body under stress. Whatever stress the body is put under, emotional, trauma, chemical or anything else, the body follows a learnt pattern of dealing with this. So the palladium allergy caused significant skin reactions on this patient. Afterwards, whatever excessive stress the patient experienced, caused a mild form of the palladium induced rash to return. It is as if the body says to itself, this is a stressful situation and I remember how I reacted to stress in the past; therefore, a mild form of the original symptoms comes back. The patient got married and the stress of the run up to this caused a mild flare up. It happened again with the illness of a child some years later.

ME and chronic fatigue

These are debilitating conditions that invoke little sympathy. Often the patient looks perfectly well and all the medical tests discover nothing wrong. It is easy to empathise with someone with a broken leg as the plaster cast can be seen, but someone who looks well, but says they feel awful, is a different matter entirely.

Functioning in normal life is either difficult or impossible for these patients. Extremes of will power are summoned just to get through the day. A pattern we quite often see is a severe infection in early adulthood such as glandular fever or a bacterial infection and a history of toxic dental treatment. Usually this condition is not alone, but comes with allergies, multiple chemical sensitivities, pain and joint problems. It can come at any age but is mainly seen in young adults. However, we have seen cases as young as eight years old and some cases in their 70s. The older patients usually are female and have extreme MCS and reactions to electrical fields as well. The basic principles of treatment remain the same. Remove the toxins correctly and support the body.

We have previously referred to the young man who became ill after his wisdom teeth were removed. Cleaning out the cavitation infections left after the wisdom teeth were removed restored his health and allowed him to finish university and find a life for himself.

CASE STUDY 15

The symptoms and causes

A young woman in her mid-twenties had been diagnosed with ME for five years. She was living at home unable to function in normal life. She had had glandular fever at the age of 19. The examination of her showed a collapsed bite due to orthodontic treatment as a teenager. She had pretty-looking teeth, but they did not fit together well, nor were they in harmony with her jaw joints; this was structural stress. She had all four wisdom teeth impacted and infected as well as several amalgam fillings.

The treatment

She went through the treatment following the basic principles as usual. We extracted her wisdom teeth and found them all to have deformed roots and were extremely smelly and infected. The memory of the smell that filled the surgery room when these teeth came out remains with us to this day years after the event. The amalgams were replaced with non-metal alternatives and the bite sorted out.

The recovery

She recovered within four months, entered university, graduated four years later and married. It was probably a combination of things that took her down, but the infected wisdom teeth were most likely the chief culprits. She be-came ill as they grew more impacted and infected. The narrowing of the jaws caused by the type of orthodontic treatment she had, premolar extraction and retrusion of the front teeth, undoubtedly restricted the normal development of the wisdom teeth.

'Sorting the bite out' is a simple phrase, but it was a very complex thing to do. It takes years of experience and post-graduate training to become competent at this. Diet and pH control is probably more important for this group than for any other as well as concentrating on gut stability. Metabolic typing is really recommended here in order to find out the correct food types, as well as keeping up a high anti-oxidant regime for life. Some sort of non-strenuous physical exercise is vital and infra-red saunas are helpful.

Irritable bowel syndrome (IBS)

This distressing and common condition has also responded to our treatment. Such cases are nearly always a combination of amalgams and infections, but there are exceptions.

CASE STUDY 16

A lady in her early 40s with longstanding IBS could never move far from the bathroom as anything she ate or drank caused a toilet visit within 20 minutes. The examina-tion showed her to have 10 amalgam fillings and a 'tattoo' area in the gum on the upper jaw. The bite was locked in, so structural stress was present as well.

Replacing the amalgam fillings, cutting out the tattoo, and sorting the bite out was enough to eliminate the IBS within two months. Sometimes a gut healing programme involving various strategies needs to be employed.

139

CASE STUDY 17

Another interesting case was the first IBS patient we ever treated. This was a lady who only had one palladium-alloy crown on a front tooth and no other dental work. The IBS started less than a year after the placement of the crown some 12 years previously. There was no evidence of infections.

The result of replacing the palladium crown was that within six months the IBS had disappeared. This was in the early days of developing our treatment protocols and it did come as a shock to us that such a simple procedure along with intravenous vitamin C could have such a profound effect.

Skin and hair

Psoriasis, eczema, dermatitis, hair-thinning and dragon skin have all responded well to this treatment. Dragon skin is not a defined medical term. We use it when the skin is very dry and scaly and shaking hands with these people feels like holding a dragon's claw. Or more accurately, what we imagine holding a dragon's claw would feel like.

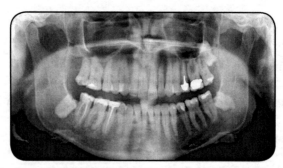

Fig. 5.1 This x-ray is from a patient with a longstanding psoriasis case with multiple allergies and chronic fatigue as well. The extraction of the impacted wisdom, root-filled and infected teeth, confirmed with a cavitat scan, and the metal crown replaced with a ceramic crown, started this patient on the road to health.

Our psoriasis patients have always had metals and infections such as root-fillings and cavitations. All the others have had either metal or infections alone or in combination. There is always an underlying gut dysbiosis that has been present for quite some time. This can be a leaky gut, inflamed gut, colon issues or underlying infection. Hair-thinning is seen nearly always in peri-and-post menopausal females. We have seen it in young women and men, but rarely. Palladium is the chief villain, but mercury and infections play their role too.

Mind, memory, anxiety, depression, and obsessive compulsive disorder

Anxiety, depression, obsessive compulsive disorder (OCD), panic attacks, irritability, short-term memory loss, brain fog, lack of concentration and loss of confidence can all be placed firmly at the door of mercury from amalgam fillings. This is not to say that infections, cavitations, root fillings and other dental metals do not play their part, because they do, but by and far the biggest villain is mercury. Remember, the largest exposure to mercury people have is from dental amalgam fillings.

Psychological issues like these can be remedied surprisingly quickly, usually in days and weeks rather than months. Sometimes, gut and allergy problems can slow recovery down; then it is a case of identifying and solving the problem for that individual patient.

CASE STUDY 18

This case is a nice one, and the patient involved ended up as one of our best and enduring friends along with her husband. All patients have to fill in a detailed questionnaire about themselves before they see us so that we can have a background knowledge of their particular issues. This allows us to allocate the correct time for the examination. The examination starts with an interview before any physical examination, x-rays etc. are done. We had allocated one hour for the interview; this was not enough.

141

The symptoms and causes

The patient was a lady in her mid-thirties, well-educated, well-read, articulate and somewhat of a challenge. The initial interview consisted of her telling us, at length and repeatedly, exactly what was wrong with her and what we should do about it.

She had had bouts of mental illness for the last 18 years and had been in and out of mental hospitals and under treatment all this time. Counselling had been ineffective as she talked and did not listen. Drugs masked the problem, but did not address the cause. The drugs she had been taking masked the symptoms and were now giving her severe side-effects. On top of this, the private insurance she had was about to stop funding any more treatment so she had to find a way out and fast. She had severe obsessive compulsive disorder, OCD, massive irrational anxiety, bouts of severe depression, panic attacks, memory dysfunction, lack of concentration, brain fog like a London peasouper and a very short fuse. Her toleration of stress was minimal. Do the symptoms sound familiar? This is classic mercury poisoning.

She had the results of a Kelmer test which showed high levels of mercury. The doctor who did the test was unable to treat her because of his own illness. As a side issue, it strikes us as a bit odd that medical doctors want to treat such patients with chelating agents but still leave their amalgams in place. A Kelmer test was very dangerous for this patient as it releases mercury into the body and it may have pushed her over the edge. We would never have done such a test. DMSA, as used in the Kelmer test, or DMPS, used as a challenge test, pull mercury out of the amalgam fillings if they are present, so both tests are dangerous and open to inaccuracy.

We did not want to treat her as she was so irrational but we felt sorry for her husband so we relented. She had eight amalgam fillings, two root fillings and a metal ceramic crown. The root fillings and crown were relatively recent and done after the onset of the illness. By a stroke of co-incidence she had kept a diary over the years. When she examined the diary she found that from her teenage years on, every visit to the dentist was followed by the onset of mental symptoms. This pattern was repeated throughout the years with the severity of the illness increasing each time.

The treatment

She went through a preparation phase and we began treatment one Monday morning. Over the next two days we removed all the amalgam fillings and took out the root-filled teeth. She was an excellent patient, nervous but co-operative. She even stopped talking, for a while at least. By Thursday midday, after the fourth vitamin C infusion consisting of 40g vitamin C with 400mg glutathione and 200mcg selenium plus B vitamins, she felt normal.

The recovery

The effect was swift, dramatic and permanent. The speed of recovery surprised even us and was due to her good lifestyle habits and good nutritional background over the years. The IBS issues took a little longer to dissipate and to this day she is intensely intolerant to wheat. She maintained the supplements we gave her to continue the detoxification for several years. This was a sensible precaution as the mercury come out mainly in the first 30 days but can dribble out for quite some time. She probably had poor mercury detoxification pathways so each amalgam filling was adding to the load and increasing her symptoms.

We wrote to her psychiatrist at length, explaining what we did and why, but he did not reply to our letter. The patient did meet the psychiatrist later on to explain to him in detail what we had done and the remarkable effects she had experienced. He told her he was glad she was well, but his interest was in the sick patients, not the well ones. He showed polite interest in her story, but he did nothing to find out what treatment had been successful for one of his patients. Could this be because there was no financial incentive in this successful treatment for psychiatrists?

We have filing cabinets full of similar cases, but this is one of our favourites due to the dramatic nature of the symptoms and the ease in which the problems were solved. To be able to help return a patient to a normal happy productive life is the greatest reward we can ask for.

Heart

I, G M-H, am the best illustration of heart problems and toxicity. I was told at the age of 28 that I had only a limited time to live and yet here I am, still here over 34 years later, to annoy the doctors. I react extremely strongly to mercury, and working as a dentist I was exposed to high levels of mercury vapour on a daily basis. I was lucky that I came across the means to control the toxicity of mercury and the knowledge of what was behind my condition. There is no trace of any heart abnormality now, all the arteries are clear and the cholesterol levels normal. I was the first to go through our treatment.

These days, I go to cardiac specialists for check ups just to show off my low blood pressure and clean arteries.

CHOLESTEROL

Cholesterol needs to be mentioned here. Over the years we have seen the same results time after time. Patients come with high levels of good and bad cholesterol. After treatment to remove their toxins, the cholesterol levels fall. The reason for this is that cholesterol is there to protect you from toxins; it wraps them up ready to be excreted. High cholesterol levels mean high levels of toxic load. The body will produce cholesterol as a protective measure. Familial hypercholesterolemia is another story, but your routine high cholesterol is there to help you. It is a sign that something is amiss; it is not the cause of the problem.

Taking drugs to reduce your cholesterol reduces your defences, which is why when cholesterol levels are much reduced by drugs, mental illness symptoms such as suicide increase, as does the risk of getting cancer. It is housewives' commonsense again. Do cholesterol reducing drugs increase life expectancy? Even the drug manufacturers admit that the drugs (statins) that reduce cholesterol levels will not make anyone live a day longer, so why bother with them?

CASE STUDY 19

My father had developed angina in later life that stopped him ballroom dancing. Getting back on the dance floor was his reason for treatment with us. We gave him infusions of vitamin C every six weeks, supplements and dietary advice.

He was back on the dance floor within 10 months. He was Portsmouth Area Champion 1942 Latin American, so you are talking serious stuff here.

He went back to his cardiologist who checked him out and discharged him as needing no further treatment. My father asked the cardiologist if he was interested in how my father had managed to recover from a condition that is generally regarded as progressive and permanent. The cardiologist gave the standard reply that he was interested only in the sick and not the well patients. Being well built, forceful and an ex-WW2 Royal Marine commando, my father physically pinned the cardiologist against the wall and told him about his route to health. The only result of this was him being banned from that specialist and hospital. He had no dental problems having lost all his teeth in the Burmese jungle in 1944. His heart problems were related to poor nutritional habits and modern medical drugs.

TACHYCARDIA AND INTERMITTENT ARRHYTHMIA

Tachycardia and intermittent arrhythmia appear to be related to oral infections and respond well to the types of treatment described in this book. These are observations we have made over the years. We may be treating a patient for something entirely different when, after treatment, the patient will say, 'Oh by the way, I never told you this before, I have had tachycardia for years but I have just realised that it is gone'. The same things have happened with arrhythmia except the patient usually says, 'I did not tell you this because (probably correctly) I thought if I did, you would not treat me, but my heart is working normally now'.

Patients with heart conditions should seriously consider that becoming toxin free, maintaining a lifestyle free of smoking and excessive alcohol, keeping up high levels of antioxidants, may offer them a better quality of life than lifelong medication might do.

Joints – arthritis and ankylosing spondylitis

Once again, the earlier the intervention, the better the result. Once damage to joints has happened, then it is irreversible, but even so, further regression can be halted. You can put the fire out, but the damage remains. This section overlaps the auto-immune section, but here we will deal with rheumatoid arthritis and ankylosing spondylitis.

The toxins that appear to have the main effect with these conditions are from infections and cavitations rather than metals. This does not mean that metals should be left in; they should be correctly removed as they exert a negative influence on health anyway, but the bacterial toxins appear to play the larger role in these conditions.

146

This is not the place to expound on rheuma factors, repetitive trauma to joints and the like; interesting though they are, it is the end result that we shall describe. Weston Price described putting an infected or root-filled tooth from an arthritic patient under the skin of a rabbit causing the rabbit to develop the same arthritic symptoms as the patient. He did this with heart disease patients too, the experiments indicating that toxin release is a factor in both conditions. It appears that Staphylococci are the type of bacteria involved, and the pH of the media they grow in will define what condition is shown. That is, some bacteria that thrive at a low pH will give one set of symptoms, but the same type of bacteria that thrive only under a different pH will give a different set of symptoms. This knowledge was discovered in the 1920s but now has been largely forgotten.

Food intolerances are very significant in rheumatoid arthritis and should be looked for. A metabolic typing test can help patients in the search for the correct foods to choose. Identifying and avoiding the worst offenders as well as maintaining high antioxidant levels are vital. Living in areas with fluoride in the water increases the risk of joint and connective tissue problems.

The cases described are ankylosing spondylitis (AK) as they had complete remission. The rheumatoid arthritis patients we have treated still have joint deformities but we have managed to either get them off, or reduce their need, for medication and further progression of the condition has stopped.

CASE STUDY 20

This was a young woman in her mid-30s. She had been diagnosed with AK two years previously. She had limitation of movement, pain, muscle weakness and fatigue.

The only dental treatment she had ever had was the removal of two impacted wisdom teeth on the right side some 12 years previously. A cavitat scan showed that the

---

147

lower right wisdom tooth area had a large cavitation infection clearly visible on the x-ray.

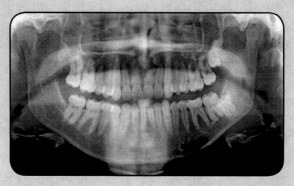

Fig. 5.2 A cavitation infection in the space where the impacted wisdom tooth had been (left side of the x-ray).

This cavitation was opened up and cleaned. It was a large hole in the bone that surrounded the inferior dental nerve which gives feeling to the lower right side of the jaw. Fortunately, the nerve was not damaged during the cleaning and the cavitation healed back to normal bone. Within two weeks, the symptoms began to ebb away and had disappeared within three months.

CASE STUDY 21

This case was much more complex and took nearly four years to complete. A young man in his early 30s and physically active became progressively more tired with muscle pains and limitation of movement. AK was diagnosed. He had two root-filled teeth which he thought may be the cause of the problem as they had been root-filled sometime before the onset of his symptoms. When he came to us, the root-filled teeth had been extracted but no change to his symptoms occurred. He had had considerable dental work done and had all the metals exchanged for composite and glass materials, all without any health benefit by another dentist. His bite was locked in and structural stresses were present.

A cavitat scan revealed infections in the bone where the root-filled teeth had been extracted, also in the lower left molar region, and underneath all the wisdom teeth. It was necessary to redo the dental restorations so that they were in harmony with the jaw joints to relieve the structural stress and this was done first. After this, all the wisdom teeth were extracted and cleaned and the cavitation infection where the teeth had been extracted was cleaned out.

This regime brought significant improvement to the patient within a matter of months. He did feel some time later that there was still infection in the jaw and a new cavitat scan confirmed this. We had to clean out the previous extraction site three times and go back into a wisdom tooth site. The new scan showed that a crowned tooth had died and this too was extracted and the site cleaned. The crown had no metal in it being made from a glass-ceramic. At each operation, a series of high dose vitamin C infusions were given. After the crowned tooth was extracted, the patient felt 'something significant had happened' and his recovery was rapid.

The probable explanation to this series of events is that although we removed a lot of the toxins and the symptoms on the first operation, one tooth was dying or dead, but this did not show on the cavitat scan or the x-ray originally. This tooth was not removed at the first operation so some of the symptoms remained. This shows the importance of rescanning and the deadly effect crowning teeth can have by killing teeth, and therefore producing toxins in the body.

One case took four months beginning to end, the other four years. In the last case it is important to note that after the amalgams and metals were removed from the mouth and after the root-filled teeth were extracted by a conventional dentist there was no change in his symptoms. The reason for this was that the underlying issue of the infections had not been sorted out and the extractions and metal removal had not been done under the correct conditions. It certainly does not mean that the root fillings, dental metals and amalgam fillings were not contributing towards his symptoms. They were all part of his toxic load that eventually dragged him down.

The key is identifying the toxins and removing them properly in the correct sequence with proper nutritional preparation and massive doses of intravenous vitamin C. There are no short cuts.

Had the patient come to us for treatment with the root-filled teeth and metals still in place, it is quite likley that his recovery would have been as quick as the young lady described earlier. Over the years, we have noticed that patients who come to us after having their amalgams and other metals removed as well as teeth extracted always take far longer to recover than patients who come to us still with the toxic dentistry in their mouths. Incorrect removal of the toxins seems to 'lock' the symptoms in place. A Swedish professor explained this to us like this, 'When the body is exposed to toxins, such as mercury or infective toxins as happens during removal, the defence mechanisms of the body are immediately mobilised. If enough vitamin C and glutathione is given intravenously at the same time to saturate the body, the defence mechanisms go into overdrive and become many times more effective than normal. Furthermore, vitamin C and glutathione safely neutralise and dispose of the toxins'.

In this young man's case he did not experience the swift release of symptoms because the previous treatment prevented this response. The young lady was more fortunate in coming to us with her toxins still in place. His case took longer to have a satisfactory result, but was still highly successful.

Autoimmune

Autoimmune means that the body makes antibodies against a part of itself and uses the immune system to attack it.

MULTIPLE SCLEROSIS

This disease has been described in the neurological section previously, but it is an autoimmune condition. The theory of why mercury is one of the causes of this condition is as follows. Mercury, because it is attracted to fat, becomes attached to the myelin sheath that surrounds the nerve fibres. This foreign particle is seen and recognised by the immune system. The immune system makes B Lymphocytes to attach to the mercury and signal to the immune system to attack it as if it was an invading bacterium or virus. The immune system attacks the mercury and the myelin sheath that the mercury is attached to causing the damage seen in MS. It is a lot more complex than this, but that is the general idea.

Other autoimmune conditions follow the same principle with metals and toxins. The genetic make up of the patient with exposure to a particular toxin will dictate what symptoms arise.

SJÖGREN'S SYNDROME

This disease fits into the neurological section as well, but it is also an autoimmune condition, so we will describe it here. We have treated a number of patients with Sjögren's syndrome over the years, all with success.

151

Sjögren's syndrome is characterised by a bewildering variety of symptoms. We do not diagnose the condition; patients come to us already with a firm diagnosis. Usually, Sjögren's syndrome patients are female, have dry eyes and mouth and many organs can be affected. There is no known cure and it is progressive according to conventional wisdom.

CASE STUDY 22

The symptoms and causes

This patient was a 40-year-old male who was very fit and athletic. Ten years before he came to us, his symptoms started with pains in his knees which slowly spread to all his joints. He was fatigued, no stamina, and he began to have limitation of movement. After eight years, his fatigue level was such that he was permanently declared sick and off work. He also had dry eyes, throat and mouth. He had constant muscle pain. He had a constant headshake, which made dental treatment interesting, and movement and severe pain in his right leg.

The previous dental treatment

Just before these symptoms started, he had both wisdom teeth extracted on the left side which took a long time to heal and was permanently painful. Two years after the symptoms had begun, he had three amalgam fillings removed without any change in his condition. The upper-right first molar became sensitive, and when he pushed the tooth outwards, a lot of his symptoms disappeared even though this tooth tested 'alive'. Three other molar teeth were root-filled and he was always 'aware' of these teeth, but no actual pain. A year before he saw us, the rest of the amalgam fillings had been removed by a conventional dentist with no improvement to his symptoms. As each year passed, his condition worsened.

The treatment

An x-ray and cavitat scan revealed extensive infections under the molar teeth in both the upper and lower jaws. We did a series of operations to remove the infections. Nowadays, we would do them all over two days, but this was an early case for us and we were overly conservative. We began on the lower left and tracked the cavitation infection from the wisdom tooth area under the two molar teeth in front. These teeth were extracted.

The uppers were exactly the same: soft infected bone around the site of the wisdom tooth extraction and the infection had spread under the molar teeth and included one of the premolar teeth. All the affected teeth were extracted.

The smell of the infected rotten bone was pungent and sour. On the right side we started with a lower molar that was root-filled and followed the infection under all the molar teeth. All the molar teeth were extracted and the bone cleaned slowly and carefully using only hand instruments.

The recovery

The symptoms lessened, but were still significant. His head had stopped shaking, his tunnel vision had cleared, the facial pains and headaches had gone, and the inflammation of the right leg had disappeared as well. The upper teeth appeared normal on the x-ray and tested to be vital or alive, but showed up as infected on the cavitat scan. The cavitat scanner does not lie. Sometimes it can show an area to be healthy when it is really infected, but if it shows that there is something wrong, there always is. All three molar teeth were removed some months later; all were infected. The wisdom tooth had rotted the bone through into the sinus and smelt, according to the patient, of old cat food. The upper-right molars were the last to be removed.

Six months after the last operation and after 20 high-dose vitamin C infusions, his symptoms cleared. He even went back to mountaineering and tried to get off the permanently-ill register and back to work.

This case showed how an infection can spread under so called healthy teeth and that the cavitat scanner is accurate. It also demonstrates that all infection has to go, no matter what it takes.

This patient lost teeth that in any normal case would be considered healthy, teeth which had never been filled. It is doubtful that he would have recovered as he did, had these teeth not been extracted. As he said, 'I will swap teeth for health any time'. There has to be good reason to extract teeth, either visual, x-ray evidence, or a cavitat scan, but when the evidence is there, it must be acted upon. Saving teeth to compromise health is not a good exchange in our view.

HASHIMOTOS THYROIDITIS

This is an autoimmune condition that disrupts normal thyroid function. We have had cases respond by removing palladium, others by removing amalgam, and some by cleaning out cavitations.

Mercury and fluoride both reduce thyroid function by direct poisoning action; if there is an added autoimmune response, it is little wonder that we are seeing the number of underactive thyroids that we do.

Most thyroid sufferers are female and have a history of early contraceptive pill use. Whether the contraceptive pill has any bearing on the health of the thyroid we are not sure, it is just an observation.

Chronic iritis

This is inflammation of the Iris. It is associated with Crohn's, lupus, rheumatiod arthritis, and ankylosing spondylitis. The standard treatment is symptom suppression by steroids or other drugs. Chronic iritis can cause other eye conditions to develop, some of which can cause visual impairment. The most common conditions include glaucoma, cataract, band keratopathy and cystoid macular oedema.

We have treated several cases of chronic iritis, all of which have responded very well to the treatment. Once again there is no known cure and it is progressive according to conventional wisdom.

CASE STUDY 23

Symptoms

This was one of our first cavitation cases treated before the invention of the Cavitat. The lady was in her early 50s and had been diagnosed with chronic iritis for three years. The condition was progressive and impaired her visual ability. She also had early onset Parkinson's-like tremor, chronic fatigue, and anxiety; the latter was hardly surprising. She had lost all the back teeth many years previously and only had the six front teeth in the upper and lower jaws.

Causes

A CAT scan, our only diagnostic tool at the time, showed dark suspicious areas in the right jaw, both upper and lower. We opened up the lower right jaw at first at the site of the first molar. I remember exposing the white sheet of bone then touching it with a drill. The drill bit into the hard, outer surface for a millisecond then jumped through into an enormous black hole. The smell was awful and characteristic of what we now recognise as a long-standing cavitation infection.

Opening the access point wider, we could see the hole stretching backwards and forwards along the jaw. The realisation of the size of the cavitation sharply increased my blood pressure and heart rate.

However, partly cleaning such a cavitation would be pointless as the infection would simply recover any lost territory after a short while. That would be like washing one hand only instead of both of them. Even after all these years, I can visualise everything about that afternoon: the smells, the feelings (the 'oh my God' type feelings), and the sights.

Treatment

So slowly and carefully we pulled the gum away from the bone and opened the bone to follow where the infection took us. The cavitation started at the wisdom tooth area and went forwards along the jaw ending up under the canine and second incisor tooth, both of which were extracted. The inner bone of the jaw (the lingual plate) was thick and held the jaw together, it was the outer bone (the buccal plate) that had rotted; this is usually the case.

We slowly scraped away the soft, dead, infected bone, a bit like treating dry rot we imagine, until solid bone was reached. The infection was not uniform in size, sometimes involving the nerve, sometimes diving through worm holes in the bone to appear further on. Some parts were as big as a hair ribbon and other parts small as string; they were always connected though. After cleaning this monster out, we washed it with saline, painted iodine and oil of cloves over it, sewed the gum back and hoped her guardian angels would be good to her.

The upper jaw was not so frightening. Here there were three separate cavitations one of which involved the canine tooth, which was extracted, and one that opened up into the sinus space of the upper jaw. Upper jaw bone is softer than lower jaw bones and has different characteristics when operating on. That does not mean upper jaw cavitations are easier to manage, usually the opposite is true. We cleaned out the cavitations, washed them, painted them and sewed the gum back over them. Quite an afternoon!

That evening, G M-H was not sure whether to book himself in for a heart transplant the following day or have a stiff drink; He decided on the latter.

Recovery

Strangely enough, there was very little post operative swelling, we had expected her to come back looking like a hamster with a bad case of mumps, but this was not the case. It certainly was not easy for her afterwards, but her eyes began to recover within the day, and after two weeks, not only had the chronic iritis gone, so had the Parkinson's-like tremor. The fatigue must have gone because one day she climbed up the four flights of stairs to the practice clutching a wooden bird house larger than herself to give us as a present. Why she chose a wooden bird house to give us is a mystery to us, but many generations of small birds have been raised in it since then.

Such operations are not for the faint hearted but no specialist oral surgeon would recognise her medical problem as being caused by cavitation infections so either we performed the operation or no-one did.

Even today, only a minority of oral surgeons will admit to the existence of cavitation infections, let alone their systemic health effect.

All the chronic iritis cases we have seen have been associated with cavitation infections and all have been female adults over 50 years old.

Glaucoma

A few words about glaucoma, even though it is an inflammatory condition rather than an autoimmune one. We say it is inflammatory

157

because the increased-pressure type of glaucoma responds well to intravenous vitamin C and high-level antioxidant supplements. This was a chance observation we noted first on Lilian's mother and found it applied in other cases as well. The non-pressure glaucoma does not respond to this treatment but the most frequently seen glaucoma is the increased pressure type.

Pain and NICO (cavitation) infections

A case illustrating NICOs has been described in the cavitation section of Chapter 3 (see Case study 9, pages 76, 77 and 78).

Unlabelled patients

Some patients are not easily categorised and so tend to slip through the medical net. Often, their symptoms change, are diffuse and hard to pin down; other times, the symptoms are varied and seemingly unconnected. All this makes it hard for any GP or specialist, no matter how competent or caring, to either label a patient or offer any meaningful treatment. We shall describe several of our most interesting and dramatic cases. The first case (Case study 24) is a doctor's worst nightmare; but the last case (Case study 27) reveals the nightmare we are living in, and we regard it as one of the most important cases we have ever done.

> ### CASE STUDY 24
> #### Symptoms
> A young woman in her 30s presented us with the following list of symptoms which she had suffered over the last five to six years. Chronic indigestion, tunnel vision, tingling and numbness of fingers and toes, loose stools, panic attacks, ear pain, facial pain over the right cheek, salty taste on right side of mouth, constant nasal drip on the right side, tachycardia, anxiety, depression, chronic fatigue and food sensitivities. She was functional and still held down a responsible job, but this was becoming increasingly difficult.

Many tests had been performed with no clear result. Interestingly enough, a course of antibiotics reduced all the symptoms temporarily. This finding is a clear indicator that infection is involved; unfortunately, antibiotics do not often give positive responses in chronic infection. We would have expected that her ESR or erythrocyte sedimentation rate (a non-specific measure of inflammation) would have been raised along with the levels of C-reactive protein, but the result of such blood tests were not available to us.

Causes

Her bite was a disaster with a mixture of amalgams, dental metals, root-filled teeth, infected teeth and cavitation infections. Her resting mercury level in the breath was 16ppm (parts per million) which went up to 101ppm after two minutes chewing gum. The limit of mercury vapour allowed in the workplace in the UK is 25ppm.

She did not have the memory loss, lack of concentration, irritability and loss of confidence which is typical of mercury exposure. A lot of the symptoms did indicate mercury exposure, but probably the main problem was infection and structural. Her body core temperature was slightly too low and her urine pH was above her saliva pH indicating a long-standing infection.

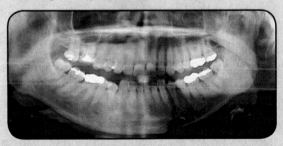

Fig. 5.3a This woman's OPG x-ray (a panoramic scanning dental x-ray).

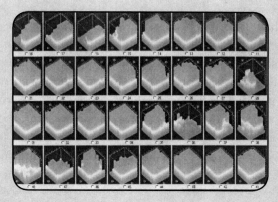

Fig. 5.3b The patient's cavitat scan.

When reading a cavitat scan, green is good (grey in *Fig. 5.3b*) and black is bad. The upper-right wisdom tooth area is 18, the root-filled tooth is 16, the upper-left wisdom tooth area is 28, the lower-left wisdom tooth area is 38, a crowned tooth is 36 and scans 45 to 48 show the teeth to be under excessive occlusal (bite) pressure.

Treatment

The x-ray shows jaw joint wear, a root-filled tooth and an odontome (a mass of calcified dental tissue) stuck in the bone between two teeth. We left the odontome where it was as there was no reason to remove it. Teeth 16, 38, 36 and 48 were extracted. The cavitation infections at 18 and 28 were cleaned out. The metals were replaced with composite and ceramic and the horrendous bite was made functional.

Replacing missing teeth was left until a later date as the main reason she came to us was to get healthier rather than prettier. In order to fill the gaps, bridges, dentures etc. could have been made and were made eventually for bite stability, but we preferred to wait until the patient has regained their health before taking this step. The treatment followed the usual course of individual supplementation: intravenous vitamin C and two days of dental treatment.

Recovery

At a check visit some months later, the patient declared that she 'felt invincible', the symptoms had gone and life was bearable again. She maintains a high level of antioxidant supplementation which she shares with her partner. When the partner began on the supplements, a restless leg syndrome disappeared after a few weeks. This shows how malnourished the population is out there.

She must have been a nightmare to her doctor, what could he possibly have done for her that made any sense at all? Every single day patients similar to her must be filling doctors surgeries with their multitude of complaints when the only answer doctors can give them is that it is 'all in your head' and offer tranquilisers and anti-depressants.

Amalgam-free?

Being pedantic sort of characters, we count how often patients think they are amalgam-free when they are not. The result is both alarming and disquieting.

Of patients who have had their amalgam fillings removed at their request, only 50% of them are actually amalgam-free. Sometimes traces of amalgam remain under composite fillings or inlays; sometimes amalgam fillings are resurfaced with composite. Crowns are often placed over amalgam fillings, a fact that just pushes the mercury along the nerves into the brain. Under a crown, the amalgam remains invisible and impossible to detect.

Sloppy practitioners are to blame as well as dentists who do not really believe that amalgam is a problem at all, so leaving it under fillings or crowns is not a problem for them. Unethical is what we would call such treatment. It appears that leaving amalgam under crowns is taught in dental schools today, it certainly was not in my (G M-H's) day, so it is the younger practitioners who are more culpable in this regard than the older ones.

CASE STUDY **25**

The symptoms and causes

A 40-year-old man, who had been healthy up to his visit to a 'holistic amalgam-free dentist' some four years previously, came to us with chronic fatigue and pain. Prior to this, his treatment had been routine. He had three wisdom teeth extracted at the age of 24, the lower-left one being swollen and painful for a long time afterwards. Tooth 36, the first left-lower molar, had been extracted two years after this, again with a history of troublesome healing. However, he had no symptoms and was functioning normally.

Being concerned with preserving his good health, he decided to have his amalgam fillings removed. He attended what he thought was the best place to have this done, but only mechanical measures and rudimentary dietary advice were used to reduce his mercury exposure. His lower-front incisors were crowned at the same time as they were slightly crooked. Acrylic (plastic) crowns had been fitted on three of the lower anterior crowns along with a bite appliance.

Immediately after this treatment, he plunged into a spell of chronic kidney pain and associated fatigue. Any dental treatment, even a scale and polish would trigger increased pain and fatigue. The left kidney was always more painful than the right. Alcohol would increase the pain in the kidneys. In his words 'the worst thing I have ever done was having these teeth done' (to become metal-free).

An examination revealed structural stress, his occlusion (bite) was far from optimum. The bite appliance made for him by his previous dentist only served to make matters worse. The cavitat scan showed that he had cavitation infections on the lower-left jaw where the extractions had been done years previously. Interestingly enough, the lower anterior crowned teeth showed healthy on the cavitat scan, but this turned out not to be the whole story. The anterior (front) teeth had proved almost impossible to anaesthetise in the past; this was a key finding.

Extensive testing had revealed no kidney problem, or any other. A nutritionist had prescribed supplementation which reduced the severity of the pain; otherwise, no form of treatment had any success. What had turned a seemingly healthy individual into a man barely able to function, with concern about being able to fulfil his job properly? The immediate cause was the poorly-designed and performed dental treatment, but this was only the straw that broke the camel's back. Bad as the treatment undoubtedly was, it only served to push him over the cliff; he was already standing on the edge.

The diagnosis of cavitation infections was confirmed by the inability of the local anaesthetics to numb up the lower front teeth. One of the properties of a cavitation infection is the ability to stop anaesthetics working on nerve blocks if the cavitation lies between the point of injection and the tooth to be worked on. Indeed, for the acutely painful NICO infections (neuralgia-inducing cavitational osteitis), this is used as a diagnostic measure to track down the exact spot where the infection is, which could be some way distant from the actual site of the pain.

For instance, if there is a cavitation at the wisdom-tooth area, but the pain was affecting teeth at the front of the mouth, usually on the same side as the cavitation, putting a few drops of local anaesthetic around and in front of the cavitation can stop the pain. This means that it is a NICO infection in the wisdom-tooth area that is causing the pain and not the painful teeth themselves, which can look perfectly healthy because they are. The dentist is often pressurised by the patient to extract the healthy teeth one after the other in a futile attempt to stop the pain.

The cavitations on this particular patient had produced toxins which, while no immediate problem, had stretched his healing resources to the limit, so the extra stress of mercury release from amalgam filling removal and the stress from the poorly constructed bite was enough to push him over the edge.

Had he had the dentistry done under the V-Tox protocols, it is unlikely in the extreme that he would have had this reaction. However, unless the underlying problems of the two cavitation infections were remedied, another stressful event in the future would have triggered some sort of health event; he was, after all, at the edge of the cliff, of which he was unaware.

The treatment

After the usual preliminaries, we cleaned out the two cavitations on the lower left jaw. His symptoms resolved almost at once by about half and his pH swung from strongly acidic to mildly acidic. A bite appliance was made, correctly, and this further helped reduce the symptoms. About three months after the cavitation cleaning, we were sitting with him reviewing the case when he announced, 'It's these front-lower crowns that are holding me back; will you take the teeth out?' The crowns were poorly done and needed replacing, but removing the teeth without a positive cavitat scan showing pathology with these teeth was a big step to consider. Detailed x-rays did show that the membrane connecting the teeth to the bone had widened and a new cavitat scan showed some stress on the teeth, but nothing dramatic.

An electrodermal test (EAV) had indicated a problem with these teeth. Not being a big fan of EAV, but trusting the patient and the equivocal results we had obtained, we arranged for the front three lower teeth to be removed. At least the teeth could be anaesthetised now that the cavitation infections had been successfully dealt with, so we took the lower-front teeth out again using intravenous vitamin C for protection. The teeth were not healthy and had a slight sour smell about them. The nerves inside the teeth were alive, but damaged when we cut the teeth in half for inspection.

The recovery

The results were astounding. The next day he came in to say that all the problems had gone, and gone completely, 'I have never felt so good' was his statement to us the following day. None of the symptoms have ever returned.

Obviously the front teeth were affecting his health a lot more than we realised and, by coincidence or not, the organs where his problems lay had Chinese medicine meridians running through them. We are not great fans of connecting teeth to meridians and organ function as the correlation can seem a little tenuous, but it worked for him. Our suspicion is that the front teeth were damaged by the plastic crowns and added to his toxic load. The cavitations were the root cause of the problem, but it required the removal of the whole toxic load to alleviate his symptoms.

We made a nylon flexible denture for him; he wanted no more crowns or bridges and said on his last visit to us that the denture functions and feels better than his own teeth ever did. That is because we made the denture to the correct physiological 'bite'. No known diagnosis, no effective conventional or alternative treatment had helped him, but identifying and the removal of his toxic load, done properly, restored his health. Life as a dentist can seldom be more satisfying than when this happens.

Addendum

As an addendum to this case, this illustrates how the treatment has to be carried out in the correct manner in order for it to be effective. He did see an amalgam-free dentist who claimed to be experienced and holistic, but the treatment he received there triggered his condition.

CASE STUDY 26

The symptoms and causes

A lady came to us from abroad; a lot of our patients travel around the world to see us. She had had a bad tremor and chronic fatigue for over 15 years. Neurologists had diagnosed 'essential tremor' and she decided to have her amalgam fillings removed. Dentists in her own country refused to believe that amalgams were the problem, so she came to England for treatment. Once again, she saw an amalgam-free holistic dentist, a different one this time, and ended up with two root fillings, metal crowns, no amalgams; her condition significantly worsened. It worsened to such a degree that she had to retire from her job, temporarily as it turned out. Once again dental treatment, this time so-called holistic treatment, had added to her toxic load and made the symptoms worse. Mercury from her amalgam fillings could have been behind her symptoms originally but incorrect removal of the amalgam fillings and the placement of metal crowns on root-filled teeth was a toxic load that was too much for her health to withstand.

The recovery

Happily, the story does end well. She did go through the whole programme and her symptoms vanished within the month and she resumed her career. Just because a patient has had their amalgam fillings replaced and are still ill, does not mean that the amalgam fillings were not behind the problem to some degree or another. It is just that the removal of the amalgam fillings may have been done in such a manner as to make the problem worse.

CASE STUDY 27

The symptoms

This case is interesting, because although the symptoms were varied and specific, no diagnosis was ever given. Indeed, the patient in question was told by eminent doctors that, 'No diagnosis means there is no illness; it's all in your head.' The patient was a bright active lady in her late 60s. She played golf, walked, cycled, took care of the house and garden after retirement, but now was unable to do any of these activities. She had had every test known to medical science, but none of the tests could reveal what the problem was. She was a non-smoker, drank little alcohol and had an excellent diet as well as taking vitamin and mineral supplements.

She had suffered from chronic pain in the right hip, muscle wasting and a loss of balance. She could only walk with support and was chronically fatigued. The symptoms had started some four years previously and had been unrelentingly progressive. She thought she had MS, but nothing to explain her condition was found by the neurologists. Her voice was getting progressively weaker and she had a constant pain in the upper-right and left jaws. All x-rays and MRI scans showed nothing wrong at all anywhere.

She had seen a holistic doctor who advised her to remove the amalgam fillings, which she did. She also had eight root-filled teeth extracted and eight cavitation operations all performed by a so-called holistic dentist. She had repeated DMPS injections, a chelator used to remove heavy metals from the body, and 24 infusions of 50g vitamin C.

Nothing helped with the symptoms, so you might assume that the doctor was wrong. Despite this expensive and massive dental intervention, no symptom had improved, just the reverse. So was dentistry behind her symptoms? Yes, absolutely and unequivocally yes. She had toxins from metal teeth, cavitation infections and root fillings for many years. Eventually her resistance to these toxins was worn down and the symptoms began.

The examination

When examined by us, she had cavitation infections in the upper-right wisdom tooth area, the upper-left jaw from the premolars to the wisdom tooth and on the lower-left jaw on an extraction site as shown by the cavitat scan. She also had one ceramic and three large metal bridges made to replace the missing teeth. One bridge started at the front incisor and went all the way back to just before the wisdom-tooth area.

The bridges had been made in a way that caused structural stress to her jaw joints and muscles. The bridges turned out to be a mixture of metals, one was almost certainly nickel-based and the others most likely palladium alloys. In our eyes, she was suffering toxic stress from the metals in the bridges and from the cavitations, and structural imbalance.

The treatment

She was not keen on losing all the expensive bridges work so recently put in so, unusual for us, we compromised. We prefer to remove all metals from the teeth and mouth before performing any surgical operation. Years of experience has taught us that metal-free mouths heal faster and have fewer complications than mouths with metal in them. Furthermore, the healing response of the patient is slowed down if they are still exposed to metals and their overall symptoms may not improve until the metals are removed properly.

Treating a patient after such intensive dental treatment is always more difficult than treating a patient from the beginning. Patients who come to us after having their amalgams and metals out, as well as root-treated teeth removed, usually require a longer treatment period to obtain satisfactory recovery. Picking up the pieces after a failed attempt at treatment by others nearly always takes longer than if we are brought in at the beginning.

We treated the cavitations first and made her an appliance to wear at night to remove the structural stress. The cavitations were both old and new and extremely large and smelly. Cleaning them out thoroughly took time and immense concentration. The old cavitations were where the wisdom teeth had been extracted some 50 years earlier. The new ones were associated with the fairly recent extraction of the root-filled teeth. Many unsuccessful operations had been done on these sites in a failed attempt to clean out the infections.

The partial recovery

Her pain in the jaw went almost immediately and some of her balance came back, enough to offer encouragement, but not enough for a normal life. Her voice was still weak.

After two months, she realised that the metal bridges had to go and we replaced them with non-metal bridges and a nylon denture.

She also had supplementation designed by us for her particular pH, maintained her own diet which the metabolic testing showed to be correct, and eight vitamin C infusions with glutathione and minerals. We also gave her extensive B vitamins and liver injections to be administered by her doctor at home. He was concerned that some of her symptoms were from functional B vitamin deficiency so some months afterwards she had the additional B vitamins. We doubt whether the extra B vitamins were necessary, but they could only be good for her overall.

After the metals were removed and the structural stress properly relieved, she rapidly recovered. The basics principles of V-Tox therapy, when applied properly, restored this patient to health and function. The best intentions of holistic doctors and dentists not using these principles had not helped her at all. For treatment to be successful it is like a dance, the steps have to be in the right order for a positive result.

The full recovery

Within a year of her first consultation with us, she could walk unaided as her sense of balance returned, her voice had come back to its original strength, her energy levels were high and she was entirely pain-free. Her muscles filled out and became defined and her posture was erect and confidant. On her visit to us, her husband had driven her from Scandinavia to see us as she was unable to fly. The trip was two days in the car and 18 hours on a ferry. Now she can fly and pops over on shopping expeditions.

She had suffered a loss of confidence mainly because of the loss of balance and relied on her husband for physical support. She remembered having started a mild irritable bowel syndrome some 25 years previously directly after the fitting of a gold crown and some unexplained health problems which were persistent, but not serious. The regrettable facts were that despite the good intentions of the doctor and the dentist, because she was not treated in the correct manner and sequence, she did not get better. When she was treated in the correct manner and sequence, she recovered quickly and fully. Indeed, she has just come by for a social call and told us, we quote her exactly, 'I am sure that I was dying when I first saw you and had I not come to you for treatment, I would have been dead by now'. Whether this is true or not, she believes it and it was nice of her to say so.

Diabetes

Diabetes is a condition we have not mentioned so far. This is an MCD that is exploding across the world. The end result of diabetes can be blindness, circulatory problems and vascular damage. It is connective tissue damage and related to excess sugar in modern diets. It was found only in the rich many years ago as they were the only ones who could afford refined sugar. As sugar has spread its malign influence across the world, so the incidence of diabetes has increased. Mercury too plays a part, as mercury from amalgam collects in the Islets of Langerhans of the pancreas that control insulin production and inhibits the proper function of the Islets.

Medical schools are researching to find the gene behind diabetes, but even if they find it, how are they going to alter the gene? Interesting, but for the patient it is totally pointless. Diabetes can be self-managed. Certainly in the early stages of the disease, effective diet modification and sensible supplementation can control diabetes and prevent progression of the condition. Amalgam filling removal which is done properly and allied to detoxification procedures such as the V-Tox therapy have shown themselves to be effective. Mike Adams'

171

book on diabetes (*www.naturalnews.com*) is to be recommended for all diabetic sufferers as it describes the diet protocols to follow.

In our experience, diabetes has proved so easy to reverse up to the insulin injection stage of the condition, that it does not warrant much comment. Once insulin injections are necessary, the progression of the condition is such that it is not reversible; but even at this stage we have seen patients that have managed to no longer need insulin injections. Diabetes is a condition of poor nutrition allowing a genetic weakness to manifest itself.

Poisoned, but no symptoms?

What makes the next case so important is that it shows that even a person that appears to be functioning at the top of his or her range, is in fact poisoned and can be made to feel and function so much better once the poisons are removed. This must also apply across the board to the population in general, who must be labouring under the effects of a toxic load from dental, medical and general environmental sources. How much better would their lives be if they could rid themselves of this ever increasing toxic load? The saving to society would be enormous as well as increasing the sum of human happiness and fulfilment.

CASE STUDY 28

No symptoms?

This case shows the magnitude of the problem we have created in this society due to toxic load from all sources. The patient is the husband of the woman in 'Case study 18' who was in and out of mental hospital for 18 years. He was a man of similar age to his wife (late 30s), no illnesses, no syndromes, no conditions and a stranger to medical treatment. He was, by all modern definitions, perfectly healthy.

The toxic load

He had 15 amalgam fillings, all fairly elderly, three impacted, but not infected wisdom teeth, no cavitations or root fillings and a good occlusion or 'bite' for once. The only toxic load we could find was from his amalgam fillings. The mercury vapour emitted from his amalgam fillings was 12ppm resting and 124ppm after chewing. It is important to remember that 25ppm is the UK limit for mercury vapour in the work place for an eight hour exposure. Obviously he exceeded the notionally safe dose of mercury vapour every single day. Dr Stock in the 1930s showed that 25ppm of mercury vapour was dangerous which is why some countries set their limit at 10ppm.

He held down a senior managerial position in a large multinational company, looked after a mentally compromised wife and was studying for an external degree that he eventually passed as a top student. He had witnessed the dramatic changes that had happened to his wife as she went through the treatment and wanted the treatment as a preventive measure rather than a cure for anything. He went through all the usual processes and ended up with metal-free teeth.

The benefits

As he said himself, the transformation on him was enormous after the treatment. He said, 'I never knew I was so tired, I have so much energy now. My thinking has become clearer and a lot faster. I have not felt this good since I was an undergraduate;'

This was a very important case as it shows how much poisoning from dental toxins the general population is suffering from. How much better would the quality of life be for the general population without these toxins? What future trouble did we prevent by removing these toxins in a safe and controlled manner? There is no way of knowing of course, but this treatment could have saved both the country and the individual concerned significant expense in medical treatment later on. Common sense really; if you put poisons into people, you can expect them to get sick.

A scientist called Richardson in 1994 showed that if an adult has four or more amalgam fillings in their teeth, they are likely to have an adverse health event due to the amalgam. This illustrates just how dangerous amalgam fillings are.

The other cases

The cases chosen are but a tiny snapshot of the cases we have treated and the records kept on file. If any particular condition has not been illustrated here, the reader can be sure that it is probable that we have a similar case in our records; for example, patients with 'electricity shooting through their jaw' or middle-aged women who sleep in tents in the garden as they cannot be near electric cables for any length of time. Space limits us here to these chosen few and for every case discussed there are other cases we could have chosen.

The variety of symptoms displayed, the age and sex of the patients is vast but the common thread that connects them all is that the V-Tox treatment worked for them. Nutritionally prepare the patients, remove metals from their teeth and jaws, remove root-filled and infected teeth and clean out infections in the bone, get the bite right, and use high-dose intravenous infusions of vitamin C with glutathione etc. Do these things in the correct order and in a thorough and correct manner, and the results can be amazing. As we have stated before, this approach does not always work, but it works in so many cases where all else has failed, that it deserves to be tried.

174

The success rate

As a broad rule the 80:80:8 rule applies. This means 80% of the patients become 80% better within 8 months. 98% of patients said they experienced significant benefit after the treatment. Some were completely better, others were not. There are no promises or guarantees with any treatment, but logic and experience has taught us that house-wives' common sense applies: if you are poisoned, you get sick.

The nature of the illness will depend on your genetic makeup, the type and amount of toxin you are exposed to, and the length of time you have been exposed to the toxins.

Opponents tell us, 'well we do implants etc. and our patients are healthy'. Really? How do they know the patients stay healthy? Do they test the patients beforehand and afterwards? Do they monitor the health of the patient? Of course they do not, they only hope their patients are healthy, they do not know or check.

In my (G M-H) case, the first symptom I would have had that something was amiss would have been sudden death most likely, dropping down dead on the street from a heart attack. Would that event ever have been associated with a reaction to mercury? Not a chance.

The plain fact is that we, as dentists, do not know if our treatment is detrimental to our patient's health. If you as a patient see the logic in what we are saying, then ask your dentist for help. If your dentist wants to continue the toxic approach of old, find another dentist who does not. Only patient pressure will force dentists to change. Change is uncomfortable as it makes us face reality and our past. This is even more uncomfortable to mercury-saturated dentists.

No placebo effect

Patients come with a multitude of symptoms and diagnoses. They are varied in age, gender, temperament, nutritional status and belief systems. The one thing that links them all is their toxic load and the fortunate fact that removing the toxic load correctly restored their health. The results cannot be placebo because their symptoms are permanently reduced or vanished. With placebo treatment, the symptoms would return in time.

175

Neither can it be due to belief. Just because a patient connects in their mind amalgam with their poor health does not mean that removing the amalgam will make the patient better because they believe it will do so. The cases show patients having removed their amalgam fillings actually become significantly worse which would not have happened if the only cause of their condition was in their minds.

Certainly, all amalgam-free practitioners will have success stories to tell, but we see their failures as well and to fail can mean a devastated life for the patient and their family. All the cases show that the correct manner of toxin removal is critical for predictable success. There is enormous personal satisfaction in seeing patients recover from what appears to be a hopeless situation.

SUMMARY

- This chapter illustrates by case histories that the fundamental cause of modern chronic disease is toxic overload.
- The name of the MCD or the label put on the patient is seldom helpful in alleviating the condition. All names and labels of MCDs are illusory because the same cause, toxic overload, underpins all of them.
- Unless proper and complete examination by knowledgeable professionals is undertaken, the nature and severity of the toxic overload can be missed.
- Even so called 'holistic dentists' can make matters a lot worse by failing to apply the V-Tox basic principles of diagnosis and treatment.
- Successful treatment is never guaranteed, but thorough and complete treatment following basic principles and a written treatment plan with good patient co-operation gives the best chance of a full recovery.
- The recovery cannot happen unless the toxic overload is identified and dealt with properly, the nutritional needs of the patient are met, and the detoxification pathways are up to the task asked of them.

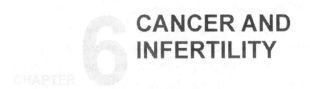

CANCER AND INFERTILITY

This chapter discusses cancer and infertility, both of which are dramatically increasing in modern society. For cancer, the emphasis is on prevention rather than cure. In order to become free of cancer once it has taken hold, it is no easy task, but usually still possible for most people. The topic of treating cancer is so large that it deserves a book on its own and will only be briefly touched upon here.

Infertility can affect both males and females and should be regarded as a modern chronic disorder rather than a disease entity. The treatment is essentially the same as all MCDs, however. Prevention programmes are for the individual who is not yet diagnosed or suffering symptoms of any of the MCDs discussed. The purpose of a prevention strategy is to make the changes necessary to avoid or significantly reduce the risk of ever developing any MCDs. This will involve lifestyle changes, diet considerations and supplements.

CANCER

Cancer is in essence no different from any other MCD. It is; however, far more serious as it is the end point of the breakdown of the body's defence mechanisms. It is more fear inspiring and is just behind heart disease as the most frequent cause of death in modern societies.

We have deliberately steered away from describing patients we have treated who have had cancer. We have done this for two reasons.

1. As the types and aggressiveness of cancers can vary so the treatment suitable for each individual patient will vary as well.
2. We do not make any claims with cancer. We treat patients who have cancer rather than treat patients for cancer.

However, what we have experienced over the years is that we have never seen a cancer develop without a chronic oral infection (a root-treated-tooth or cavitation infection) being present. Treating cancer without addressing the oral infection only allows the cancer to return in the future. Treating a chronic oral infection once the cancer has started is not enough; specific anti-cancer therapies have to begin as well. This is a contentious statement but we are not alone, as will be shown, in finding this out.

The rate of cancer has increased dramatically over the last 100 years from 1 in 30 to now 1 in 3 of the population. The cure rate is only 5% better than 50 years ago according to a recent report in the New York Times, despite all the hype surrounding the issue. Developing a personal prevention strategy is a far more sensible thing to do rather than try and play catch up after the onset of the disease. All cancer treatments are complex, expensive and time consuming whether they are conventional or alternative or a mixture of them both. The outcome of any treatment regime is always uncertain so it is sensible to reduce your own risk of the condition so that you never have to face the fear and anxiety that a diagnosis of cancer always produces. Having some knowledge of what to do if ever faced with a cancer diagnosis is useful too. The fear inspired by the diagnosis of cancer can paralyse coherent thought and the patient can be pressurised into treatment that is unsuitable, unnecessary and even harmful to them.

What is cancer?

Cancer cells are primitive; by and large they are misshapen cells that have an anaerobic metabolism rather than the normal aerobic metabolism. Anaerobic metabolism functions without oxygen and is only 18% efficient compared to aerobic metabolism. Cancer cells have a different electrical polarity to healthy cells as well. They can be considered to be the body's response to damage which has gone hideously wrong and out of control.

The causes of cancer
GENES

Cancer is a genetic disease. The type of cancer a patient contracts is due to their genetic makeup, but this does not mean that because you have a cancer gene you will get cancer. What it does mean is that in order to turn this cancer gene on you will need to be exposed to a specific toxin for a specific period of time with a lowered immune response due to diet and other causes. Only if all the boxes are ticked will the disease start. Having a cancer gene means that it is possible for you to have the cancer, but it is not inevitable.

CHRONIC INFLAMMATION

Cancer is not a condition that magically started suddenly one day. Like all MCDs, it is usually the consequence of many years of exposure to toxins with an inadequate nutritional diet. Remember what we stated in the beginning that all the cancer patients we have seen have had chronic dental or oral infections.

The parents of cancer are allergies and chronic inflammation. The long-term effect of these is to wear down the immune system. When the immune system is overloaded for too long, it can let down its guard and instead of ruthlessly disposing of defective cancer cells, it allows them to live. Consider the micro-environment where a cancer starts. Chronic inflammation creates an acidic environment in the body and the body responds by trying to control the pH by dissolving the bones releasing large amounts of free calcium. A toxin of some description, be it chemical or a bacterial exotoxin (a toxin excreted by a microrganism), reaches some tissue and damages that tissue. The body will try and repair the damage, but in a low-oxygen and low-pH environment with an overloaded immune system surrounded by free calcium, the repair message is distorted and a cancer develops. There is, of course, a little more to it than that, but that is the basic reason behind the development of most cancers.

179

DENTAL INFECTIONS

Dr Hans Nieper, a German oncologist, stated that dental infections, especially the condensing osteitis (inflammation of the bone) seen around root canals, was a leading cause of cancer. Dr Robert Dowling of the North Carolina Institute of Technology goes a step further. He states that all cancers start with a dental infection. He goes on to say that thermal imaging or identifying heat sources in the mouth can pinpoint where the infection is. Not only that, but the side of the face where the infection is will dictate what side of the body the cancer will start on. For instance, a right-sided infection from a cavitation or root filling will give breast cancer on the right breast. Similarly a left-sided infection will give cancer on the left breast. If there are infections on both sides then the cancer will affect both breasts. Therefore, if the cancer is treated, but the underlying mouth infection is still there, it is only a matter of time before the cancer returns. This applies to all cancers, but is perfectly illustrated in breast cancer.

This is certainly a contentious statement that would be dismissed by medical cancer specialists and the majority of the dental profession as arrant nonsense. However, that would only be their opinion as there is no scientific data as yet to base any firm conclusion on. Over the past 30 plus years of experience as working general dentists, we would agree with Dr Dowling completely. This does not mean that all dental infections such as root fillings and cavitations will always lead to cancer. It means that we have never seen a cancer patient who does not have a chronic dental infection in his or her mouth and that the side of the infection mirrors where the cancer is in the body.

CASE STUDY 29

Here is a typical example of what we find. The patient had brain cancer on the left-side of the brain. The Cavitat scan showed infection around the last two left-upper molar teeth, where the wisdom tooth had been extracted years before. The upper-left first molar had been root-treated two years before the start of the cancer.

180

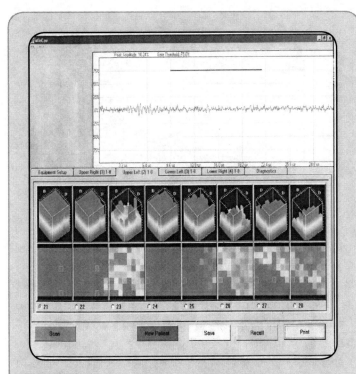

Fig. 6.1 The cavitat scan.

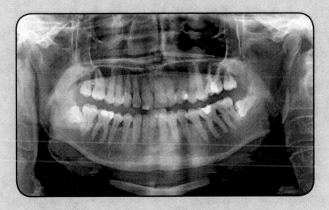

Fig. 6.2 The OPG x-ray.

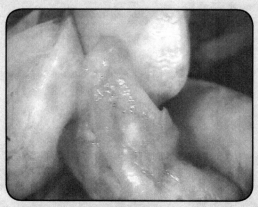

Fig. 6.3 The large, soft, infective mass attached to the roots of the extracted root-treated tooth.

When the root-treated tooth was extracted, it had a large, soft, infective mass attached to the roots *(see Fig. 6.3)*. In fact, this tooth had five roots instead of the normal three roots. The x-ray looked as if the tooth had a perfectly normal well-executed root filling in place *(see Fig. 6.2)*. The extra roots were hidden from the x-ray and would have been full of dead, rotting tissue. There was no way the dentist who performed the root filling would have known about the extra roots, he did what he thought was correct. Even if the tooth had only three roots, there would most probably still have been dead tissue in the lateral canals that would have rotted and produced toxins.

In this patient, the tooth behind the root-treated tooth was infected. After extraction, the cavitation infection in the wisdom tooth area was large enough to stick a finger in. Whether removing these infections will allow the patient to beat the cancer is always unknown, but it should certainly give her a better chance of recovery and if she does beat the cancer, removing the infections should reduce her chances of a reoccurrence later on.

Preventing cancer

Cancer cells develop in all of us all of the time, but they are identified and dealt with by our immune system. A fully-functioning immune system is your best, indeed your only, defence mechanism against cancer. A compromised immune system can be overwhelmed by the onslaught of cancer cells produced by the body. Coupled with the cancer cells' rapid duplication as well, a cancer becomes established. By the time any overt symptoms of the cancer are noticed by the individual, it will already have been in place for several years.

The obvious steps to take when trying to recover from any type of cancer are similar to those already explained in this book. Remove all identifiable toxic loads correctly and support the immune system in every conceivable way. Do this by eating the diet right for your metabolic type, sensible supplementation with antioxidants, minerals, appropriate amino-acids, moderate exercise, and avoid all toxins from whatever source. Make sure you keep an optimum pH in the body; do what you can to flood your body with oxygen.

DIET

Meat eaters are supposed to have an increased risk of cancer, especially over vegetarians. Even this is misleading as the definition of red meat in the studies included processed meats, cured meats and commercial hamburgers, all of which are far removed from clean, fresh, grass-fed, antibiotic and hormone-free meat.

Once again there is no one-size-fits-all as metabolic type 2s will increase their risk of cancer on a vegetarian diet as they will become more acidic on a purely vegetarian diet, G M-H being a classic case in point. It becomes further complicated as we see metabolic type 2s actually require a vegetarian diet usually at the beginning of a major detoxification regime as can be seen on their individual metabolic test before going back to the type 2 animal protein diet.

Cancer treatments

The difference between cancer and other conditions is that cancer is usually more serious. It can be considered the end point of the disease journey not just a stop on the way. Recovery, if possible, will take

183

longer and require more effort and resources than other conditions. There are numerous strategies available to treat cancer and it is not within the possibilities of this book to either list or comment on any of them. However, despite the seriousness of cancer it is essentially the same as all the other conditions described in this book and the successful treatment of it follows the same principles.

WHICH TREATMENT?

We never said any of this was easy and it is an example of where open-minded experience shows its true value. The trouble is that the average patient is left totally alone in a minefield of opinions, many masquerading as facts, with little guidance to find their way through. Many of the so called 'experts' have their own agendas and commercial priorities to fulfil not to mention arrogance and misguided self-belief. This applies as much to the alternative field as the conventional. There are good people out there on both sides of the fence, but do not take anyone at face value. It really is hard for the patient to know who to believe and what the appropriate treatment is for them as an individual.

Cancer statistics

Cancer statistics are misleading and should be viewed with scepticism. For example, a recent study from Italy showed that over 60% of cancer patients undergoing conventional therapy were also having alternative treatments but were not telling their doctor about the alternative treatments. Since the doctors do not know all the treatments the patient is receiving, how can they possibly know which treatment really is effective or not? For any meaningful results you would have to separate those who have had conventional treatments from those who have not; from those who are trying both conventional and non-conventional treatments at the same time; from those who have proper diets for their type with appropriate supplementation and sugar elimination from those who have the standard western high sugar, low nutrient value diet; from those who live in a water-fluoridated area to those who do not. (There is a 13% increase in the risk of contracting

184

cancer because of the fluoride, according to Dr Dean Burke, former chief scientist at the National Cancer Institute).

Success or failure?

Reduction in size of a tumour is often described as success but as one patient of ours recently put it when told that chemotherapy had reduced the size of his tumour, 'I have still got the tumour so what sort of success is that?' The survival rate quoted for various cancers is also increasing. However, that is due more to earlier detection of the cancer than actually living longer.

Logically, the only true measure of success is total elimination of the cancer and the patient still being alive to tell the tale. Death is the endpoint for measuring success or failure of any cancer treatment, anything other than this is just nonsense. Some cancers have a good five-year-survival rate in the traditional view, but the usual treatment leads to leukaemia (a different type of cancer) after seven years. How does that appear on the statistics? Success or failure? We would regard that as failure not success, but it is not how your average oncologist would view it.

Our recommendations

Our recommendations concerning cancer are simple.
1. Have an effective prevention strategy to significantly reduce your risk of cancer.
2. Find out enough about conventional and alternatives treatment regimes so that you already know what treatments to avoid and what treatments to follow should you ever be unfortunate enough to find yourself faced with a diagnosis of cancer.

The type of cancer that develops is dependent on the genetic make up of the patient and the nature of the toxin produced by the bacteria. In treating cancer, whether by chemotherapy, radiation, surgery or any of the myriad of alternative therapies, unless the source of the cancer, i.e. the chronic dental infection, is removed successfully, the chances of the cancer returning at some future date will be increased.

From a personal point of view, we believe that supporting the immune system by all possible means makes more sense than damaging it with poisons as in chemotherapy or burning it away as with radiation. The success rates of both these treatments are depressing and the long-term damage to the body caused by these conventional treatments can reduce the chance of any sort of non-conventional treatment being successful. Just because a treatment is non-conventional does not mean it is a successful treatment. No-one has all the answers and some of the advocates of alternative treatments can be as narrow-minded as their conventional counterparts. This is yet another reason to do your research into the facts before you are faced with treatment decisions rather than be rushed into something unsuitable.

The dental infection theory applies even to those who have had all of their teeth extracted many years prior to the onset of their cancer. Extracting teeth without thoroughly removing any underlying infection around the teeth will lead to cavitation infections in the bone which are symptomless. We have picked up many such 'silent' cavitation infections in patients years after the extractions were done.

Cancer is a complex issue but most cancers can be prevented and a high proportion of cancers can be successfully treated if sensible and logical steps are taken. It is a minefield for any patient to enter, as they are exposed to competing and conflicting information and it is easy to be led into expensive, ineffective and even damaging treatment. Finding experienced practitioners that can offer sensible advice and treatment strategies is no easy task.

INFERTILITY

This is an issue that can affect both males and females. A good starting point when considering this issue is Mike Ziff's book, *Dental Amalgam, Infertility and Birth Defects*. This book uses referenced scientific data to confirm the link between dental amalgam, specifically the mercury released from amalgam fillings, and infertility and birth defects.

The increase in infertility now experienced by society is due in part to social changes such as the later age couples attempt to have children, but largely due to the increase in toxins in the environment from all sources and the lower nutritional value of the food we eat. A strong, relaxed mental attitude is needed as well. Positive thoughts about conception and birth are far more constructive than concentrating on why one is not conceiving. Just think about the babies born to couples who have just adopted a child after years of trying and failing to conceive. Once they relax and concentrate on the new child rather than focusing on why they are not conceiving, conception becomes easier.

Pottenger

Diet plays a vital role in infertility. The importance of diet was amply illustrated by Pottenger and his cats in the 1930s. Pottenger kept cats as experimental animals. Some of the cats ate nothing but cooked food whilst others had a more mixed diet. Some cats were fed on pasteurised milk alone and other cats had raw milk alone. Breeding from these cats was normal for the first generation. Both conception and births were normal. However, this changed in successive generations. Each group of cats was bred within the group. The normally-fed cats had normal births and offspring in each generation. The raw-milk cats likewise had each successive generation normal in every way. Not so the cooked-food and the pasteurised-milk groups. In these groups, after the second generation, conception became increasingly difficult until by the fourth and fifth generation, the cats had become infertile. Each generation showed physical deformities that became more emphasised with each generation. These deformities included longer thinner limbs, smaller jaws with crooked teeth and smaller hips. The cats were increasingly more violent and aggressive to such a degree that the last generation could only be handled wearing protective clothing.

The smaller hips meant that giving birth became ever more difficult with many cats dying in the process of parturition or giving birth. The difference in body shape and behaviour between the sexes became ever more blurred to a point where the young were androgynous. Interestingly enough, this degeneration was reversible up to a

point. The cats took a couple of generations on a mixed diet to revert
to normal, but there was a point of no return.

CATS AND HUMANS

The comparison between these luckless cats and today's generations
is startling. The youth of today are taller with longer limbs, there is an
epidemic of small jaws and crooked teeth and the difference in body
shape between the sexes is reducing, a fact noted by Weston Price in
the 1930s. It should come as no surprise then that both conception
and giving birth is more difficult to accomplish for this generation
than their predecessors.

Whether we are experiencing an increase in aggressive and angry
behaviour is open to question, but certainly the young appear more
disassociated from society in general than ever before. Pottenger's
experiments illustrate the vital importance of diet, the effect of which
may not be seen in the current generation. *The result of the cat's diet
was a steady decrease in the ability to conceive.* The increase in infertility we are experiencing now could be partly the result of what
we have done to our food since the advent of chemical farming

Mercury also plays a pivotal role in both aggressive behaviour
and in infertility and birth defects. As the greatest source of mercury
to humans is from dental amalgam fillings, it is this dental toxin that
is to blame. Mercury can reduce both female and male fertility rates
quite dramatically.

Female fertility rates

A study of dental nurses showed them to have a fertility rate only
50% of normal if they worked for a dentist who used amalgam. Spon-
taneous abortion is three times higher in female dentists than normal;
not only that, they have more difficult labour and a higher death rate
of the babies after giving birth.

The same result has been seen in many animal experiments after
exposing the animals to mercury. Monkey experiments show that
mercury reduced the number of live births, but caused no overt signs
of toxicity in the offspring. Other animal studies clearly demon-
strated not just reduced fertility rates, but that 26% of babies died

188

compared to 1% of controls after exposing the pregnant animals to mercury. To put it unequivocally, the mothers exposed to mercury appeared entirely normal, but more of their babies were born dead.

The menstrual cycle

Disturbances in the menstrual cycle will naturally alter the fertility rate. Exposure to mercury caused hypermenorrhea (heavy and long lasting menstruation), excessive blood flow, irregular intervals and painful menstruation. The longer the time of exposure to mercury, the greater the chance of a problem. The rate of anovulation (failure to produce a viable egg) is nearly doubled in those exposed to mercury compared to a control group.

The thyroid

Another fertility problem is the action of mercury on the thyroid. We have seen that mercury is preferentially absorbed by the thyroid where it depresses thyroid function. In time, the damage to the thyroid becomes irreversible. Thyroxine from the maternal thyroid is vital for the brain and neural development of the baby.

Alcohol increases the absorption of mercury vapour, depositing the mercury in the mother's thyroid and in the thyroid and liver of the foetus. This means that mothers who drink alcohol during pregnancy increase the amount of mercury deposited in the unborn child from their own amalgam fillings.

Endometriosis

Endometriosis is thought to be an auto-immune disease brought on by a disturbance of the immune and hormone system. We have previously described how mercury alters the immune system. Endometriosis is a common cause of infertility, up to 40% of all infertility is put down to this disease. Due to the action of mercury on the pituitary, adrenal glands and progesterone production, mercury from amalgam fillings is regarded as a significant factor in endometriosis.

It is best to avoid replacement of amalgam fillings during pregnancy as removal of amalgam may increase the amount of mercury in the body. Alcohol should also be avoided. It is important to remember that the foetus throughout the whole time of its development is exposed to mercury from the mother's amalgam fillings.

Male infertility

Over 50% of infertility problems are caused by a fault in the male sperm. The fertility of men is significantly altered by mercury. Mercuric compounds were marketed in England from 1938 as a spermicide, (a substance that kills sperm). It was very effective, although G M-H's mother would claim otherwise!

Heavy metals including mercury, gold, aluminum and vanadium have been found in high concentrations in sperm. The motility and the speed of the sperm is reduced by mercury compounds. A man is considered sterile if 25% of his sperm is abnormal. Mercury inhibits the production of DNA in the sperm, DNA is the carrier of genetic information. RNA synthesis is also inhibited. The function of both DNA and RNA are complex to say the very least but the alteration of the production of these genetic messengers by mercury is likely to mean reduced male fertility. Animal experiments have confirmed this.

Selenium is absorbed into the sperm. Indeed it is so important to the sperm that if selenium is in short supply in the body, the testes get priority for existing supplies. Mercury is also stored in the testes where it readily combines with the selenium thereby reducing the amount available for healthy sperm production.

Accidental industrial exposure to mercury over an eight-hour period caused impotence lasting many years. This does not mean mercury from amalgam can have a similar effect, but just to show what a powerful long-term effect a small exposure to mercury can have on the male reproductive organs.

BIRTH DEFECTS

Mercury from a mother's amalgam fillings has a pathological effect on the development of her foetus and if the baby is breast-fed, the baby will receive mercury after it is born as well. It takes two days for the mercury leaking from a newly-placed amalgam filling to be deposited in the foetus. Maternal milk concentrates the mercury so its level is four to eight times higher than in the blood. Mercury passes through the placenta unhindered. One function of the placenta is to prevent toxic material from the mother injuring the foetus. Mercury is so biologically active that the placenta presents no barrier to it.

All mercury is not the same

Mercury vapour, as given off by amalgam fillings, is absorbed up to 50 times more in the foetus than any other form of mercury. Also, inorganic mercury, i.e. from amalgams, was 12 times more likely to go through a placenta than organic mercury from food. Indeed, mercury from food like fish does not increase the foetal mercury level. This means that the developing baby absorbs more mercury from its mother's amalgam fillings, more aptly named as mercury implants, than from anywhere else. So, if there are any fish left in the ocean, we guess it is safe to eat them in moderation.

The damage to the child

So it is clear that mercury from amalgam is deposited in the foetus, but how much damage does it cause? During pregnancy, the levels of mercury in the mother rises by nearly 50%. The numbers of still births as well as live births, but with defective babies, have a direct correlation to the level of mercury. Mercury and cadmium were also found to be factors in reducing foetal nutrition to a degree that death, congenital abnormalities or growth retardation in the baby were possible. Mercury also damages the blood brain barrier of both mother and foetus. It can even enter the brain directly from amalgam, by-passing the blood brain barrier and infiltrating the nerve cells. This means that the brain is prevented from absorbing the vital nutrients needed for full and proper development. Very small amounts of mercury, less than one part per million, cause this effect.

The enormous consequences of this will be made clear. The mother with an average number of amalgam fillings absorbs more mercury into her and her baby's body on a daily basis than was used in the following experiments. The results were confirmed by two animal experiments and the changes were permanent. The higher the amount of mercury absorbed, the more the learning capacity was reduced. Mercury reduces the intelligence of the child, the higher the mercury level, the lower the intelligence. As mercury is absorbed into the brain and central nervous system throughout the development of the baby, this can result in functional disturbances and behavioral alterations later in life. The research subjects exhibited marked hyperactive behavior.

It gets worse, lead and mercury act synergistically; this means that together they have a greater effect than the same levels do alone. Lead also reduces intelligence and is present in our environment.

It should now be crystal clear to everyone, apart from those in charge of dental undergraduate training, how dental treatment, specifically amalgam fillings, can reduce fertility in both sexes as well as increasing the risk of a defective child.

Any couple who are considering having a child or are having difficulty with conception should not just have the amalgam fillings removed but all metal fillings removed correctly and safely.

Caution: Going to a local dentist who does not use the full precautions required to protect the patient during mercury removal when having the amalgams replaced could make matters worse. Seek out a knowledgeable, committed dentist for this sort of work.

SUMMARY

- Cancer is a genetic disease, but our experience shows that there is a direct link between a chronic oral infection and cancer.
- Cancer is the same as all other MCDs, but it is more serious and takes a more complex approach to recover from than other conditions.
- Cancer is the end point where the body's defences have given up.
- It is easier, cheaper and considerably less traumatic to prevent cancer rather than attempting to cure it.
- The increasing infertility in modern society has its roots in poor nutrition and increasing toxic load.

7 PREVENTION STRATEGIES

This is really basic stuff and should not come as a surprise to any-one who has persevered so far with this book. The three components of prevention for all MCDs are the following.

1. Nutrition;
2. Toxic load reduction;
3. Lifestyle modifications.

1. NUTRITION

The overall goal is to have your body at the correct pH with enough vitamins, minerals, and amino-acids to function at its optimum; sim-ple, but not easy. Metabolic typing is the next logical step. This will guide you on what foods to eat and what foods to minimise in order to create the best pH condition in your body.

Water

The next point is water; clean pure water. You must be sufficiently hydrated with clean water for any body system to function well. By water we mean water not tea, coffee, beer, cola or soda drinks. The quantity of water to drink will vary from individual to individual and the conditions they place themselves in, but as a general rule anything from 0.75 to 2 litres of water a day is good; drinking more than this can be counter productive.

Tap water, because of the chlorine and other contaminants, is not suitable for drinking. Filtering tap water before drinking is a good idea as this removes most of the impurities, but there are several points to consider. The filter must be in good condition. By this we mean not too old so that the effectiveness of the filter is reduced and not contaminated by bacteria growing on the filter. It must be a good filter to start with as not all filters are created equal. Reverse osmosis filters are very efficient but can leave the water acidic and strip out the good mineral content of the water as well.

Distilled water is completely stripped of minerals as well as taste and requires energy input so it is not carbon friendly. The latter two should have minerals added to them before use.

Water systems that separate the water into acidic and alkaline variants by electrolysis have become increasingly popular. The idea is that the acid water is thrown away and the alkaline water is drunk. The technology is too new for any long-term judgement to be made; the systems may well have some merit, but the units are expensive to buy and also need power to function so they are not carbon friendly.

The water should not be too cold either as this has the effect of a brake on the digestive system. Sipping very hot water is a Tibetan therapy for chronic disease; very pleasant as well.

Supplements

A high antioxidant intake is essential. Oxidative damage from free radical attack leading to chronic inflammation and then onto MCDs must be avoided and where it occurs, repaired. The key is enough antioxidants. Diet alone is not enough in our polluted world as we are all under increasing oxidative attack from the toxins in our general and personal environment. The degeneration in the quality of modern food means that food alone cannot provide enough vitamins, minerals and antioxidants.

Supplementation of vitamins and minerals is essential.

When choosing supplements, care has to be taken to separate the wheat from the chaff in the quality of any supplementation undertaken. Supplements should be in a natural form rather than a synthetic form as this will increase their effectiveness and the rate of absorption.

194

Any predisposition to an MCD has to be taken into account. For instance, if heart disease is a family weakness, it would be sensible to increase vitamin C, vitamin E, vitamin K, Co Q10 and serrapeptase enzymes. If neurological conditions are the family weakness: dementia, Alzheimer's, Parkinson's etc., then extra alpha-lipoic acid, B vitamins in all forms and L-carnitine over and above the base level of anti-oxidants would be the way to go. Auto-immune conditions such as multiple sclerosis or myasthenia gravis may require Dr Klenner's regime of B vitamins, choline and magnesium. If it is cancer that runs in the family, then vitamin D with vitamin A, iodine and selenium may be worth considering along with glutathione complexes. Vitamin A comes with a caution against overdosing as vitamin A is damaging at too high a dose, being fat rather than water soluble. The same applies to vitamin D. Professional guidance is advised before deciding a supplement regime.

ANTI-INFLAMMATORIES

Breaking up an inflammatory process is obviously vital and essential fatty acids (EFAs) are required. These are the omega 3s, 6s, and 9s oils taken in the right proportion. There are excellent proprietary brands that offer the correct blends or you can take your own mixture. Hemp oils, flax oils and fish oils are what we are talking about. The only care you need to take is to make sure that the fats have not turned rancid which means they have been oxidised. This can happen in some capsules and is very easy to detect by the smell of an open capsule.

CASE STUDY 30

In order to illustrate what we mean, this is what I, G M-H, take on a daily basis and have done so for many years. Heart disease is the family weakness and at 28 years old the official diagnosis was irreparable heart damage leading to early death. That was 35 years ago and not only am I still here, I have not seen a doctor for professional reasons for many years.

Daily intake: VTP3 (this is a typical mixture given to our patients), but at half dose. Full-dose VTP3 contains 4g vitamin C, 200mg glutathione complex, 75mg methionine plus most of the minerals mentioned below.

In addition to the VTP3 powder, I take the following.

Vitamin C	10g to 20g
Vitamin E	800iu
Beta-carotene	30mg
Evening primrose oil	500mg
Co Q10	200mg
Vitamin D3	1200iu
Selenium	200mcg
Flax oil	1000mg
Alpha lipoic acid	250mg
Vitamin B complex	50mg for most of the B vitamins
Multi-vitamin	one capsule
Multi-mineral	one capsule
Calcium AEP (vitamin M1)	300mg
Magnesium AEP	200mg
Magnesium oxide	500mg
Chromium picolinate	200mcg
Zinc	15mg
Serrapeptase enzyme	30mg
Boron	3mg (prevention of osteoporosis)
Saw palmetto	900mg (prevention of prostrate problems)
Soya lecithin	2400mg

Chronic obstructive pulmonary disease (COPD) can be relieved with serrapeptase as can other degenerative heart conditions. However, after trauma or those with high blood pressure, caution must be observed. Also, since the majority of soya is now GM we do not recommend soya lecithin as a general supplement. It does have protective abilities in coronary artery conditions. Furthermore, soya lecithin has oestrogen mimic properties which can play havoc with some people, be warned.

This list is given only for illustration purposes and is not a recommendation. It is what is needed for G M-H with his familial or genetic weaknesses and lifestyle. It may not apply to you. The cost for such a regime is about the same as a pack of cigarettes on a daily basis. It may look like a lot of supplements to take and it is a lot of supplements to take, but it must be borne in mind that G M-H is exposed to mercury vapour on a daily basis removing amalgam fillings. He has a hereditary predisposition to heart problems and reacted extremely strongly to mercury with a Melisa test. Even with all the precautions taken in the practice such as air filtration, mercury absorption masks and so on, G M-H will have some contact with mercury vapour at work. If cancer was the family weakness, we would have added 3g B17 (laetrile) and more glutathione to the list. If it was MS and the like, we would have increased the vitamin Bs and the calcium AEP. If cognitive degeneration was in the family, then L-Carnitine would have been added and so on.

Where to buy supplements

Since no two individuals are the same, neither are two supplement regimes the same. However, the general principle of high levels of anti-oxidants and minerals should always be adhered to. In the beginning, deciding on what supplements to take, how much of each and where to obtain them can seem a little overwhelming. Expert independent advice can be sought and the internet will provide a lot of information.

Many supplements are sold on a multi-level marketing (MLM) basis which can lead to overenthusiastic, uninformed selling. Some MLM products are excellent, others less so. Our advice when buying supplements is to be cautious and ask questions.

Sugar

Sugar intake in all forms must be reduced. This will eliminate most processed foods and soda-type carbonated drinks from the diet. Sugar is cheap and used virtually everywhere in food manufacture. Sugar feeds cancer par excellence.

Salt

There is a lot on nonsense written about the harmful effects of salt. What should be written is that refined table salt is really harmful, but natural salt such as unrefined sea salt or Himalayan salt has many positive health benefits. Indeed, one gram of Himalayan salt taken with one gram of vitamin C up to five times a day can be used to treat deep-seated infections such as Lyme's disease.

Fats

Do not be fooled by the low fat frenzy currently in vogue. Everyone needs fats, but good fats, not trans fats. Eat butter only, not the margarines which are an industrial product. Do not be taken in by the cholesterol myth either, even the conventional doctors now admit that they have got that one wrong. Get enough good fat on a daily basis.

Red meats

These are the current *bête noire* of the alternative health community. Once again, this is only partially correct. Yes, red meats do promote cancer; however, it comes down to the definition of what are red meats. The red meats that are dangerous are the processed meats, the burgers and similar industrial food. Included in this group are the corn-fed beef cattle as their fats are changed. Whole red meat from

198

a clean source, including the internal organs, has a positive health benefit, especially for the right metabolic type individuals (such as G M-H). The animal should have been grass-fed if beef or otherwise have lived an outdoor life. Raw foods should be eaten wherever possible for the high enzyme and vitamin content and it goes without saying to avoid chemical additives. These include artificial sweeteners, monosodium glutamate, food colourings and preservatives such as nitrites in meat etc.

Organic food

Food sources should be as clean as possible without making a religion out of it. By this we mean organically sourced if feasible, but this is not always possible, so do the best you can to reduce chemical contamination of your food. For instance, this can mean soaking vegetables in food grade 3% hydrogen peroxide before use and removing the outer surface or peel as that is where most of the chemical residues can be found. Food is for enjoyment and positive social interaction. Food should not be a source of anxiety or guilt. Do the best you can but if circumstances are not ideal then accept the fact.

2. TOXIC LOAD REDUCTION

This will entail careful scrutiny of all personal care products such as deodorants, toothpastes, cosmetics, shampoos, sunscreens and the like. All such products are available in forms that are not harmful to you. As a rule of thumb, anything that is advertised is a chemical concoction to be strictly avoided. Advertising costs money usually at the expense of the quality of the ingredients. A little research on the internet will show you what a wide choice there is of non-toxic personal care products available so that you will not have to expose yourself daily to a variety of man-made chemicals and scents. Such chemicals and scents can cause problems from allergy to dermatitis and cancer and you can live nicely without these!

Air

The air you breathe can be cleaned, a little, by wearing personal ionisers around the neck in polluted places. Aircraft, for example, are confined metal tubes with low-oxygen-content recycled air that is likely to have jet fuel fumes incorporated into it. Wearing a personal battery operated ioniser in such a situation makes travelling less risky to your health as well as a more pleasant experience. The ioniser emits charged particles which clears the pollutants in the air. A graphic illustration is putting an ioniser in a glass bowl full of cigarette smoke and seeing how quickly the smoke clears.

Never use man-made scents or perfumes and never, ever use the room freshener plug-ins. Volatile organic carbons (VOCs) are a potent source of cancer and these artificial scents contain VOCs. It is no coincidence that the longer you spend indoors, the higher the risk of cancer and other illnesses. Ever wondered why this is? Ventilation and removing the object of any odour is far better than trying to cover it up with another smell.

Medical and dental toxins

Have your dental toxins removed correctly and carefully examine your medical drug intake. The aim would be to eliminate or at least reduce the intake of all types of medication. You may need to seek advice from a sympathetic and knowledgeable health professional for this. Less is always better when it comes to dental and medical treatment.

Cleanses

Consider colonic cleanses. This can be accomplished by diet and oxygenated magnesium supplements or colonic irrigation. When considering the latter, the effect can be dramatically positive, but you must have it performed by a skilled and experienced operator without using any pressure apparatus. Enemas can be done at home; the use of an enema board is helpful in avoiding an unnecessary mess. A variety of herbal mixtures can be used in the enemas and coffee enemas are especially good at relieving chronic pain and supposedly removing liver toxins via the portal vein. Kidney cleanses should be performed

200

before liver and gall bladder cleanses. There are both gentle and more radical cleanses available so what is used is up to the individual and their own unique circumstances.

Starting off gently is always a good idea. There are many cleansing recipes available and we are not going to discuss the pros and cons of each one here. The first time a liver flush is done is a salutary experience when you see what has actually come out of you. Personally we do these cleanses once a year, but do an anti-gut parasite cleanse twice a year. We use an electronic gadget from Russia called, appropriately enough, Sputnik that emits harmonic vibrations after swallowing. This removes all parasites. Quite a few patients have undergone this treatment and collected the parasites to bring in to us for observation and discussion.

There are herbal and chemical anti-parasite regimes as well, but these take quite a long time and perseverance in order for the regimes to perform correctly and most people do not take them to the end. It is probable that for a healthy, developed immune system, you need exposure to various gut parasites at certain times in your life, but keeping their numbers down every so often definitely has enormous health benefits.

3. LIFESTYLE
Alcohol, drugs and cigarettes

What we mean by this is avoiding doing certain things and encouraging you to do others. For instance, avoid tobacco in all forms. Give up smoking and avoid secondary smoking. Avoid all recreational drugs at all times for ever. A recreational drug alters your brain chemistry, otherwise it would not be used. This is never positive and can have permanent consequences on your mental performance and state. Alcohol should be used, not abused. Organic wines and beers are way ahead of their commercial cousins in flavour and taste. Even if too much is drunk, the after-effects are not as severe as the chemical commercial concoctions so widely advertised and marketed. Sensible use of alcohol can have positive health consequences, especially red wine (due to its antioxidants, especially reservatrol), but red grape juice has the same health benefits. No-one needs alcohol daily, so think before you drink is the order of the day. Spirits have no positive benefits at all, but G M-H is being hypocritical here as he has a collection of over 50 different malt whiskeys and does not keep them for the pretty shape of the bottles. However, this is not a religion, so the occasional indulgence can be tolerated.

Exercise

Exercise is vital and whatever form it takes to suit you is good. The only bad exercise is too much exercise which can lead to oxidative stress and tissue damage. You should take exercise in a form which you enjoy otherwise it becomes a chore and will eventually be abandoned. Exercise is better performed as a group activity as there are social interactions to be experienced playing sports rather than lonely miles on a treadmill or pounding streets breathing in car exhaust fumes. Exercise should be fun and it should be regular. We have known severely disabled patients visualise exercise. For example, they imagine running down a sandy beach along the waterline and feeling the texture and temperature of the sand and sea as well as the sun on their backs. This has both physical and psychological benefits for the individual.

Positive mental attitude

This leads us nicely on to the development of a positive mental attitude. Do not invite bad things into your life. If you concentrate on the negative side of things, your cup is always half-empty never half-full, you will create the condition you are concentrating on. *Molecules of Emotion* by Candice Pert already says that if you are immersed in misery, you will create the cellular receptors that will reinforce this feeling of misery. Likewise if you are happy and positive, you will have more happy and positive cellular receptors. A biological validation of sorts of the Law of Attraction. This law states that what is foremost in your mind is what you will attract to you. A variation of this is what my mother (G M-H) said years ago, 'Be careful what you wish for because you will get it'.

202

This does not mean you should whistle gaily through life without a care even in dark times. You can never appreciate the light unless you have experienced the dark after all. It means that you can take control of your life even in only small chunks at first, and build on this. You are in control of your life even if you do not realise this immediately. This realisation can lead you to health.

Sunshine or helios therapy

What utter nonsense has been forced down our throats about the dangers of sun exposure. Sunlight makes vitamin D and the majority of the population is chronically short in vitamin D. Lack of vitamin D increases the risk of cancer dramatically as does slapping on sun blockers and creams. Most commercial sun creams and oils are far more carcinogenic than excessive sunlight and must be avoided. Sun exposure gives you cancer is the message but the protective creams and oils are far more dangerous to health than moderate sun exposure. Commercial values triumph over commonsense values yet again. Use the less toxic sun creams that are available if you need them at all. Personally, we have found that with a high level of anti-oxidants in the body, we can stay out in the sun without burning for a long time, but obviously this will vary from individual to individual, so care is the watchword here.

This is an example of medical fashion. One hundred years ago, helios (sun) therapy was recommended and special clinics were established for patients to expose themselves to the healing properties of the Sun. Now the Sun is our deadly enemy to be avoided and blocked out while we smear ourselves with carcinogenic chemicals.

PLANNING

As ever in life, the answer lies in the middle, not at the extremes. Any individual developing a prevention or treatment strategy against an MCD, as the two are very close to each other in many regards, must not rush into anything. It is a topic to be discussed with a partner and the family in order to arrive at an achievable and comfortable result.

Much thought should be given to every aspect of nutrition, toxin reduction and lifestyle issues before making any plan.

Remember, such a plan is a plan for living not a bolt-on addition to be discarded after the fashion changes. As such, great care and thought should go into the development of a prevention strategy, but the pay off is a healthy, long and active life. There can be no greater reward than this. Mind you, going to the doctors for them to search rigorously and find nothing wrong with you is pretty cool too!

SUMMARY

- Prevention strategies should be thought about and implemented. These will consist of diet, supplements and lifestyle changes.
- No-one can do it all, so do what you can without feeling guilty about what you may have missed. Just taking 2g Vitamin C along with a multivitamin and mineral every day would substantially lower your risk of contracting a lot of severe conditions.
- A positive mental approach is a great help as well.
- Nutrition, toxic load and lifestyle have to be examined with honesty.Permanent changes may have to be made.
- Seek agreement with partners and families before implementing changes.
- Let food and drink be a source of pleasure, not a source of guilt and anxiety.

8 YOU ARE UNDER ATTACK

The reasons behind how this sorry state of affairs arose are explained in this chapter due to special interest groups and the nature of political decision making. How and why you are under attack is explained and advice on how to protect yourself and your family from the attack is offered.

SCARE TACTICS

A patient of ours, a sensible middle-aged grandmother, once told us, 'When you go to the doctors you are under attack. They put scare posters on the wall to frighten you into having vaccinations and when you see the doctor all they want to do is force drugs onto you.' This was after her own experience where prescribed statin drugs for her 'high' cholesterol had severe side-effects causing her to stop this medication. Because of a hiatus hernia (acid reflux) she had developed a few years previously, she had to stay on other drugs to ameliorate the symptoms of the hiatus hernia or get cancer of the oesophagus (her doctor's words).

After we had removed her amalgam fillings and infected teeth under the V-Tox protocol, her cholesterol level dropped. Taking apple cider vinegar with honey has also stopped the hiatus hernia so she no longer needs the drugs. Her faith that the health system was there to help her was shattered. 'They wanted me on these drugs forever without ever finding out what was really the matter.' Taking responsible informed action is a positive step that should keep her alive and healthy for a long time.

She is, of course, right. We are all under attack and it is up to each and every one us to protect ourselves from the attack; no-one else is going to do it for us, it is just the way the system works. This is not a criticism of the western medical and dental systems, more an observation.

SPECIAL INTEREST GROUPS

We are under attack from all the special interest groups that control and influence political decisions at all levels of government. It is the same for the medical and dental fields as it is for everything else. Provided you are aware of this, it is possible to live a reasonable life and protect both yourself and your family from the worst excesses of these special interest groups.

When patients come to us, they complain about being abandoned by medicine and dentistry, about the feeling of being alone, that no-one is out there to help them. It is really that they have just come to the realisation that the 'cradle to the grave' care that they were led to believe was available from society and theirs by right, is just an illusion, a noble idea but not attainable. It has never been attainable; you are and were always responsible for yourself. It has suited some of the special interest groups to foster this illusion of cradle to grave care, but at the end of the day, you really are alone and responsible for your own wellbeing. The real question is how it ever became like this, a topsy-turvy system that pays lip-service to health, but actually encourages disease. Who is to blame and what can be done about it are the next questions.

Politicians

Politicians are easy targets, but the blame is shared between the professions, the media, the pharmaceutical industry, and the agro/chemical and energy industries. Politicians are seldom experts in any field and in order to deal with the perceived problems of the day they seek advice from experts. Indeed, they are open to fierce criticism if they do not. Unfortunately, the experts come from the special interest groups who claim to have the expertise in any particular subject. These experts serve the special interest group to which they owe their livelihood, status and sense of belonging. They do not serve the interests of the public or the planet at large. The experts often claim that they serve the interests of the public and the planet, but it is patently obvious that most of the time they do not.

How it works

The public are prepared by media exaggeration about the latest scare, be it SARS, bird flu, swine flu or whatever. The problem is made apparent and the solution, in this case vaccination, is proposed and big money is to be made. The politicians have to follow the hype or be accused of failing the public; massive public funds are given to drug companies and research institutions to develop and manufacture vaccines. The media would destroy them if they did otherwise and the media is aware of its paymasters. Just witness all the drug advertising that is omnipresent in all forms of media in the USA.

SARS came, killed a few hundred people, created a massive media scare, $800+ million dollars were made available for research and nothing more was heard of SARS; then it's on to the next scare and the next big pay day. All these industries are driven by profit, not ethics, and there are many examples of this, some of which we will get to later on. Provided we know this, we can protect ourselves from them and their agents.

GM food

A perfect example is the GM food industry. The GM food industry claims that GM technology can feed the world, whereas the truth of the matter is that there is already enough food to feed the world, it is the distribution system which has failed.

The point of GM food is to feed the bottom line of the balance sheets of the companies involved and nothing else. It really is a Pandora's Box they have opened and no-one can foresee the end result. The purpose of GM trials is to spread the genes as the pollen from these plants carries for miles beyond the containment area, once the genes are 'out there', the companies believe we will be forced to let them have their way.

GM crops require more chemicals than non-GM crops, that is the primary reason they were made. The company that owns the patents on the crops also makes the chemicals the crops need.

The politicians, generally being scientifically illiterate, are easy targets for the propaganda of the GM industry. Added to which is the financial muscle of the companies (politics is an expensive business after all), the media manipulation of the suppressed results of the harmful effects of GM, and you have a perfect illustration of a special interest group at work.

Think-tanks and organisations with innocent sounding names are created and financed by the industry in the hope of giving the industry's version of GM third-party credibility. Outright bribes to politicians have also been made by GM companies to allow production of GM crops in an effort to get around regulatory processes; some of these bribes are public knowledge.

Other industries

Such behaviour is not exclusive to the GM industry, but it is widespread throughout the major industries. The development of the electric car was hindered by the auto and oil industries as they believed such developments would hurt their profits. Companies exist to make a profit and nothing more. This is neither right nor wrong, it is just a fact.

They can think no more than the next earnings quarter where the stock market demands that they make increased profits. The bonuses, the salaries, even the jobs of the executives are on the line, so the long-term good of the many (and the planet) is put to one side for the short-term needs of the few.

The pharmaceutical industry

The pharmaceutical industry is also a good example of a commercial special interest group. The profits of the drug industries depend on disease, not the promotion of health. In fact, western medicine depends on disease for its finance, not the maintenance of health and the history of western medicine is one of promoting the interests of the drug companies.

208

The recent Viox scandal where a drug's side-effects, which included death by cardiac failure, were known but suppressed so that the company that made the drug could make millions in profits. It all came to light after a conservative estimate of 50,000+ deaths. The fine the company paid was small in comparison to the profits made on the drug before it was withdrawn. This means the incentive for repeating this with other dugs is still there. Unfortunately this is not an isolated case. Profits before ethics is the rule not the exception.

VACCINATIONS

Vaccination is another example of profit before ethics; do vaccines actually work? If you go behind the published statistics and look at the evidence, the effectiveness of vaccines is called into question, to put it mildly. The typical claim of the vaccine producers is to say that in the last 20 or so years the incidence of a particular disease has been reduced and this is due to the introduction of vaccines. The actual figures look impressive until you realise that the incidence of the disease was reducing at the same rate or quicker than before the introduction of the vaccine, and in some cases, the introduction of the vaccine actually increased the incidence of the disease in question. Mark Twain's quote of 'Lies, damn lies and statistics' comes to mind.

Doctors make money with vaccines. Even in a socialised medical system such as the NHS in the UK, the doctors get paid bonuses if they vaccinate the majority of their patients. Vaccines can be damaging in themselves; Gardasil, an anti-cervical cancer vaccine, has killed several hundred girls now and injured many more and it is only effective against certain selected types of cervical cancer. Is it worth the risk? Were the girls involved told of the risk? What is the cost/benefit ratio? The answers are not available as it is a commercially sensitive area for the company. They are even trying to push it onto boys now to 'prevent transmission of the virus' without any data to properly show that it would be effective. The vaccine is only effective for two years and only needed by the sexually active, so why is it promoted for 12-year-olds other than for pure profit?

The flu vaccines are preserved by Thimerosal. This is a mercury containing preservative that is extremely toxic. It is being withdrawn from other vaccines, but it is still in the flu vaccines. The safety studies on Thiomerosal were performed in the 1930s by giving it to terminally ill patients who were only a few weeks away from death to see if they died more quickly. They appeared not to die more quickly, so Thimerosal was deemed safe. This is absolutely true, you could not make this up if you tried, it is beyond the imagination of any rational being.

A study of old folks' homes in north-eastern USA showed that residents who had the flu vaccine were more likely to contract Alzheimer's than residents who did not have the flu vaccine. Considering the biochemistry involved discussed earlier in the book this was to be expected.

Another sobering fact is that the flu vaccine is made against last year's flu virus, not this year's type; the whole exercise appears pointless apart from the significant financial considerations.

Vaccination is the holy writ of medicine as fluoridation is for the dentists so no criticism can be made against it by any doctor without an extremely high risk of being subject to massive retribution by the governing authorities; ask Dr Andrew Wakefield. As an aside, an Australian doctor working with the Aborigines found that vaccine damage to children could easily be reduced. He discovered that if a child had low vitamin C levels in the urine due to a cold or other infection, the chances of a vaccine-damaged child were increased markedly. Waiting until the child had normal vitamin C levels in the urine prevented the vaccine from damaging the child. The vitamin C was necessary to protect the child from the toxic properties of the vaccine; simple, cheap and effective. So why is this not standard medical practice? Is it because it is connected with vitamins which seems a bit fringe medicine or is it unknown to the average doctor as such a test would show patients that vaccines can be dangerous?

CANCER

There has been approximately every six months since 1968 (as long as G M-H can remember) a 'breakthrough' against cancer announced by some drug company or set of researchers. Even so the rate of cancer rises remorselessly. The latest breakthrough announcement is that oxygen kills cancer. Otto Warburg told us that in 1935 so either someone is not reading or it is yet another spurious 'breakthrough' announcement.

The cancer industry is huge; it employs thousands of people. The turnover for chemotherapy drugs is measured in billions and the cancer charities are amongst the richest charities in the world. That means that there is very little financial incentive to actually find a cure or method of preventing cancer. President Nixon poured billions of dollars into the war on cancer only for the researchers to tell him that the war was lost and the money gone.

The constant media announcements about an imminent cancer breakthrough serve several purposes, however. It lets the paying public believe that something is being done and soon they will be saved from this modern scourge. Cancer has always been around, but never so prevalent as in today's society. It also keeps the money flowing to the companies. Why do the cancer charities not sponsor research into therapies that have been reported to help cure cancer? Therapies such as intravenous vitamin C, B-17 or laetrile, low-dose Naltrexone, ozone, Coley's Toxins, Essiac, Budwig's Protocol, enzymes etc. We could name over a dozen more. You would have thought that the charities would research into any reported help for cancer but they do not. The money only goes to support research into existing methods and theories of treatment. The answer can only be that it does not suit the purpose of these charities to actually find a cure for cancer. You can draw your own interpretation on that. Indeed, any therapy that may threaten the accepted norm of chemotherapy is ruthlessly dealt with. This is well-documented and does not need expanded upon here.

The media duly dishes up the 'breakthroughs' without ever questioning its validity or veracity or even the source of the announcement. The news of the 'breakthrough' is usually from the public relations department of a drug manufacturer promoting their products anyway or to keep the funds flowing. The media knows who its paymasters are and is under severe financial pressure these days due to competition from the internet so it knows better than to question the sources of its information. Eye-catching headlines are good for business.

The professions

The professions are also a special interest group. The dental profession operates a closed shop policy and the medical profession would like to, indeed it does have a closed shop policy in several parts of the world. This means that only registered qualified dentists can practice dentistry and considering what is involved that is a very good thing. You would not want your aromatherapist to start extracting your impacted wisdom teeth after all; that would be an invitation to disaster.

A profession operates a closed shop policy, in theory anyway, to protect the public. However, it also serves to protect the interests of the members of the profession as well as acting as a brake on scientific progress. Which comes first is open to different opinions. The consequence of a closed shop is control over the members of the profession. Should any member step out of line, he or she can be expelled from the group and their livelihood is gone. This is a great incentive not to rock the boat and keep things the way they are.

The medical and dental professions are supposed to be scientific disciplines and evidence-based. As new knowledge comes to light it should be seamlessly integrated into the healing arts for the benefit of all. Plainly, this is not the case. The majority of medical treatments are not scientifically-based anyway according to the *Lancet*. Take mercury amalgam as a filling material and fluoride for examples from the dental profession. There has been enough reputable science published about the harmful effects of mercury released from dental amalgam that the scientists in the field wonder why this material is still allowed to be used.

To quote Prof Boyd Haley, 'Arguing the case against amalgam with the dental authorities is like arguing with the town drunk, no matter what the evidence you have, you end up nowhere.' Professor Vimy goes even further, he says, 'The dental authorities that still allow amalgam to be used are either incompetent or corrupt, there is no other explanation.' Both are leading researchers in the field.

212

Fluoride

Fluoride has become religious dogma to the dental profession. Water fluoridation has become accepted in large parts of the English speaking world and it is acknowledged dental policy all over the world that water fluoridation is a good thing despite the evidence against it. Well, it is good for dentists, as dentists who work in fluoridated areas earn more than dentists who work in non-fluoridated areas. Work that one out!

In Europe, a more pragmatic approach to water fluoridation has been taken. In areas where it has been tried, it was found to be ineffective and withdrawn, for example Basel in Switzerland. The politicians of the European mainland are also mindful of being accused of forcing mass medication on the populace, the atrocities of the Second World War being still fresh in their memory; for mass medication is what adding fluoride to water is. This contravenes the Nuremburg Convention. If the dental profession was evidence-based and mindful of the science, why is amalgam not banned and the water-fluoridation policy abandoned?

Politicians who seek advice on dental health matters will naturally ask the dental profession for this advice. Politicians are unlikely to know enough about dental health themselves which is perfectly normal. A politician cannot support a clean water campaign when the 'experts' in the field are against him, the media would crucify him unless public opinion is massively in favour of clean water. Since the media is fed the positive spin about water fluoridation and it will not search out the facts for a variety of reasons, the public are misinformed about the real consequences of adding fluoride to water (increased cancer risk etc.). The public think fluoride is good, the 'experts' and the media tell them so and it would be remarkable if the politicians did not follow suit. The fault lies squarely with the dental profession which has made water fluoridation a religious dogma in spite of the evidence. The pity is that the religious dogma of fluoride is hidden behind a mask of supposed science.

THE PROFESSIONAL AUTHORITIES

The general dentist is less at fault than the authorities over him. Dentists do what they have been taught to do. Questioning the status quo is a dangerous business. Dentists do things to teeth and doctors prescribe drugs. It is the way things have been taught and the way dentists are paid.

You do not get promotion within the dental hierarchy if you step out of line, so the individuals who wish to rise through the ranks into positions of decision-making have an incentive to keep things as they are if they wish to keep the status, lifestyle and money promotion gives them. All the research money and effort goes into making what already is, better. Change is permitted only if it is within the existing accepted framework. If scientific facts show the framework to be faulty, it is best to ignore the uncomfortable truth if you want a quiet life.

Dental academics and others have told us that they want 'No change on our watch'. This means that such individuals know the truth, but are self-serving rather than interested in the truth and as such are basically corrupt. The same applies to medicine as well. The revolutionaries or heretics, we have been called both amongst other less flattering titles, are burnt at the stake. Only when the old guard dies out and are replaced, can new ideas be accepted. Their successors claim the revolution for themselves and rush around giving each other prizes. That is how most areas of science progress; it is not honest, but it is the way things are.

> 'It is difficult to get a man to understand something when his job depends on not understanding it.'
>
> Upton Sinclair

The media

It gets worse in that public opinion is media-led and the media is easily manipulated by special interest groups. Added to which, the attention span of the public and the media is so short today that even if the tide of opinion is against you, all you have to do is wait for the spotlight of attention to be directed elsewhere. A British civil servant

214

who was the chairman of an EU committee examining the safety of amalgam told us that no matter what we find (about the harm amalgam does) all the committee has to do is wait a few days until the public attention is diverted elsewhere, then carry on as before. He meant he was going to give amalgam a safety approval rating no matter what. We managed to stop him, but that is another story.

There is no possibility today of a newspaper campaigning against a drug like Thalidomide as the Sunday Times did in the 1960s. Today's newspapers would not keep the story alive long enough for the authorities to be forced to take action. Gossip about celebrities or the latest reality show results take precedence. The media has been effectively neutered.

> **Note:** The key fact in all of this is that the politicians will follow public opinion, but only when public opinion is overwhelming and clear. In all other cases, politicians will follow the opinion of the special interest groups. Special interest groups are concerned about themselves, not the public at large or the planet.

HOW TO PROTECT YOURSELF FROM MODERN MEDIA, MEDICAL, DENTAL, AND INDUSTRIAL EXPLOITATION

Ignore the media

The media is not there to inform you so that you can make sensible informed decisions about your life. The purpose of the media is to serve the purposes of its (very few) owners and paymasters. It seeks sensation, immediate gratification of feelings to prevent thought, *Schaden Freude* at the plight of others, and manipulation of its audience instead of the truth. If you are aware of this, then you are less likely to fall under the influence of media manipulation.

You will soon see the scare tactics at work. It could be swine flu, for instance, to get you to swallow a useless antiviral drug or get vaccinated with an experimental vaccine. What the media did not inform you of is that vitamin D and vitamin C are the safest and most effective

215

way of both treating and preventing swine flu. But then no-one makes big money from non-patentable vitamins and there are no sensational scaremongering headlines for the public to feed upon.

> 'I do not take a single newspaper, nor read one a month, and I feel myself infinitely the happier for it.'
>
> Thomas Jefferson

This is excellent advice and is equally correct now as it was 200 years ago. The same applies to TV and radio news programmes, do not tune into them. The constant drip feeding of all the negative items is not conducive for a healthy mental attitude and, let's face it, you do not need to know about the child murders and similar items in far away places that do not concern you. None of it is real news anyway, it is 'news' for manipulative purposes.

Soap operas are equally as bad. They thrive on conflict, but in a highly dramatised form that does not mirror everyday existence. They encourage the belief that such dramatised conflict is normal in life and are excellent vehicles for opinion manipulation. Soap operas are there to fill in time, sell ideas and goods and prevent reflective thought. Ignore them totally. They are a form of television Prozac.

Ask questions and research all possible solutions

Severely limit your use of all medical services to the absolute minimum. If you are offered a drug, always ask the following.

- What condition do I have?
- What is this drug supposed to do?
- How long do I need to take it?
- What are the side-effects?
- What are the alternatives?

If you do not receive good answers, then seriously consider whether taking the drug is really in your best interest. Always ask questions. If the doctor thinks you are being a nuisance, change doctors.

216

On a personal basis G M-H has not taken a prescription medicine for so long he cannot remember the last time, certainly 15+ years and he is old enough to remember when Winston Churchill was Prime Minister! Do your own research, you may be surprised at the result.

TRAVEL VACCINES

Take travel vaccines for example. We have travelled to all sorts of different places over many years without having any vaccines and without catching any diseases, apart from one from an over-friendly snake; the same applies to Malaria.

We did some research and came up with various strategies for preventing these conditions without using drugs. We are not recommending anyone *not* to have the travel vaccines or malaria prophylactics; that is a personal decision, but we did not want to risk the side-effects of the treatment which are frequent and uncomfortable.

To date that has been highly successful for us. One of our patients travelled through Cambodia, Laos and Vietnam for over two months with a young family. They refused the vaccines and drugs, but took instead some homeopathic remedies, iodine, grapefruit seed extract, tee tree oil etc. and never had a single medical problem of any description. This was in stark contrast to the others in the group who had followed the traditional western medical advice. Drugs and vaccines are toxins and we want to reduce our exposure to toxins. 'Poisoned people get sick' is the theme of this book after all.

Politicians cannot help

Politicians cannot protect us as they are influenced by the special interest groups, and for the public, one set of politicians is much like any other set of politicians. In an election, the public are asked to choose between Tweedledum on one side and Tweedledee on the other; it makes by and large very little difference to their lives which one is in power hence the public apathy with voting in democracies. It matters to Tweedledum and Tweedledee personally who is in power, but to no-one else.

The special interest groups back all political groups just to make sure they are on the winning side so they do not care who wins and

217

the public know that they will be paying no matter who wins so they do not care either. An approach of co-operation rather than competition as proposed by the Zeitgeist movement does seem infinitely more sensible for the future of the planet and its inhabitants, but we live in the now and have to deal with the reality of our situation.

WHERE WESTERN MEDICINE EXCELS AND FAILS

Western medicine is at its best in acute or trauma conditions. If you are cut out of a car wreck, you do not want the paramedics to deliver you to your homeopath. You need the casualty specialists to keep you alive and the orthopaedic surgeons to put you back together. Usually this works very well, but they missed G M-H's broken neck which happened after a high-speed motorcycle crash on a race track. The broken neck was found by a NUCCA therapist, Heidi Grant, in London some 20 years later and confirmed by x-ray. The neck vertebra is held together with connective tissue.

Chronic and degenerative conditions are entirely a different matter. The doctors are only partly to blame. Their whole education and indoctrination is drug-based, not nutritionally-based; indeed, traditionally the doctors have been very hostile to nutrition; you only have to witness the hysterical attacks against vitamins over the years to realise that. The system the doctors work in does not encourage anything other than the traditional drug-based approach and the penalties for bucking the system are draconian.

The public share the blame as well. They have been educated or indoctrinated to expect a drug when visiting the doctor; indeed, unless they go away with a prescription in their hand, they feel somehow cheated. The doctor is, or should be, a medical advisor, not the conduit for medication.

The public at large is waking up to the reality that they are indeed alone and under attack. Their mistrust of politics and government is at an all-time high and increasing. The sheep-like acceptance of medical dogma and practice is slowly dying as the gap between the propaganda and reality is perceived and experienced.

GENERAL ADVICE

We live alienated from nature, no longer do we live as part of it. The further we move away from nature, the worse it will be in all aspects of existence for all of us. If you hold to the conspiracy theories, this is all part of the plan for control. Conspiracy theories are good fun and some may even be true, but they are irrelevant. If you live a life of your truth, teach others by example, and do not buy into manipulation of media and the other special interest groups, you will have an excellent chance of a healthy, worthwhile, and fulfilling life. Do not struggle or fight the system, use love and example to create the changes you want instead.

OUR POSITION

We do not fear personal or professional attack. For us, the truth, as we have discovered it, is the most important factor to live by. We cannot and will not deny it, come what may. For one thing, we are old enough to have created a situation where we can live comfortably without working, so removing our licence to practice holds no fears. We work, with a passion, because we know we can make an enormous difference to people's lives by creating the conditions that allow them to heal.

SUMMARY

- Special interest groups manipulate and control the media and political decisions.
- Special interest groups serve their own needs, not those of the public. They may claim to serve the public, but this is arrant nonsense.
- Media 'news' and 'soap operas' are vehicles of public opinion manipulation and control.
- To protect yourself, take nothing at face value. Ask questions and do your own research. It has never been easier to do this thanks to the internet.
- Live your truth and lead by example.

CHAPTER 9

WHAT DO I DO NOW?

DENTISTS

If, as a dentist, you have reached this stage of the book and not had an apoplectic fit or died of rage, then you will be one of the select and growing group of dentists that have realised that the way we were and are trained is inadequate for the future needs of the patients we serve. Having come to that life-changing realisation, the question is always asked, 'What do I do now?' and there is no easy answer.

Self-assessment

It starts with taking a look at yourself and your situation both personally and professionally, an inventory if you like of your skills, the gaps in your knowledge and the type of practice you are in now. From this you can find out what you need to learn and search for places to glean the theoretical and practical skills you will need.

Perhaps the most important task is the one most often neglected; that is to write down what your professional (and personal goals) are. Unless the goal is written down, it is only an aspiration or wish, the goal has to be written down and referred to regularly. This constant reminder helps provide the motivation and discipline that is required on the hard road ahead.

What type of practice do you want, what kind of patients, where do you want the practice to be and so forth. These are some of the questions you need to ask yourself. In other words, where do you want to be, when do you want to be there and what steps do you have to take to achieve this? Do not expect to find the answers all at once, neither will the answers always be the same which is why you need to write it down and refer to it regularly.

Peer pressure

Do not expect it to be easy either, certainly now in the beginning of this dental revolution, for that is what it is. Some of your professional colleagues will treat you with scorn, amusement and fear, but always with a grudging respect for you are going where they cannot imagine. Mind you, it is hard to initiate any sort of change from a comfortable status quo and even harder if you are severely mercury toxic as are most practitioners.

When we go to 'regular' dental gatherings, as soon as it becomes known who we are, we find ourselves standing alone with a 12-foot space all around us. It is as if our ideas are contagious and an unspoken quarantine zone must be established to prevent a new idea from escaping. It is of course quite ridiculous, but an indication of the fear that new ideas generate.

New training

One of the learning paths will be to come to us so we can show you what we do. We give training to small groups and certification can be achieved in our methods. As the groups grow, then new knowledge and techniques are shared amongst the group members. We do not claim to have all the answers and we are always open to better ways of treating our patients.

The reason for the certification process is to protect the patients. We have trained dentists before, but the problem has always been that the dentists shortcut the treatment protocols. They were not prepared to do the full examination, nor individualise the supplementation. They gave everybody the same minimum amount of vitamin C in the infusions and did not always remove the metals in the mouth. This produced mixed results, as you can imagine, and it is the patient who is the loser. They expect to receive the full healing treatment, not a shortened version designed to increase the dentist's earnings per hour. When we certify dentists, the patient can be sure that the dentist has received all the training and support from us that is possible in the V-Tox therapy, but we cannot be certain that the dentist will not shortcut the process. However, we do check up on the dentist and any falling short of the mark will have the certification removed and we will personally sort the problem out for any patient.

Dentists should become members of the International Academy of Oral Medicine and Toxicology (IAOMT) and possibly the Biological Dental Society or other mercury-free dental societies. These offer moral support from like-minded dentists and spread the knowledge and experience around.

MEDICAL DOCTORS AND ALTERNATIVE PRACTITIONERS

Medical doctors may be able to diagnose in part dental toxicity, but they can only treat the symptoms, not the cause of the problems. Time after time, we see patients who have been extensively and expensively treated, sometimes for years, by a succession of doctors, specialists and alternative practitioners, but all they can achieve is, at best, some amelioration of the symptoms for a limited time.

Certainly, improving the diet, intelligent supplementation with enhanced digestion and colonic function will improve the overall wellbeing and health of the patient; but unless the underlying dental toxicity problems are dealt with properly, the patient will never be able to fully recover his or her health.

Testing

Doctors and others do perform expensive and multiple testing, but as we stated earlier, a sick patient gives a sick patient's results. Testing performs three useful functions.

1. It is a good fee earner.
2. It lets the patient feel something is being done.
3. It protects the practitioner in the event of legal action against them by either the patient or a professional body: GMC, GDC, State Boards, etc.

222

The cancer patient with the brain tumour which we referred to earlier (page 180) is a case in point when it comes to medical intervention. She has had conventional and alternative treatment for over eight years with this tumour after a variety of medical tests and the best she has achieved is a slowing of the growth of the tumour for a while. Since the underlying dental toxicity problem of the root-filled infected tooth and the cavitation infection were not addressed, all the money and time spent on treatment and tests has been largely wasted. We performed some specialist tests after the infection was dealt with which pointed out the way treatment might be successful.

Hammer and nail

But the doctors do what the doctors do. If you have a hammer, every problem is a nail. If a hammer is your bread earner, then anything that stops you hammering is a distinct and personal threat to you and your chosen lifestyle; it is a threat to your social status and ego. Hence one of the reasons for the aggravation we dental and medical mavericks have to overcome during our professional lives. Doctors and alternative practitioners in the main do not realise the severity or the prevalence of these dental toxicity problems; and even if they did, they can do nothing about them.

Remember the psychiatrist (page 144) and the cardiac specialist (page 145) of earlier chapters. There is little incentive for the doctors to send the patient to a trained dental practitioner for the removal of dental toxins for fairly obvious reasons.

An ideal world

What should happen, of course, is that the doctor takes charge of the case and co-ordinates the healing. He can send the patient to the dentist for examination (in order to assess the dental toxins), arrange the supplementation, the intravenous infusions and the follow-up care. He can, and should, instruct the dentist to remove the identified toxic problems and make sure that the best interests of the patient are served. Alas, this is Utopia; what a fulfilling professional life it would be for both doctor and dentist if such relationships were a regular occurrence. The doctor could then actually care for people as they wanted to do

223

when they entered the profession rather than act as a front man for the pharmaceutical industry. The dentist can display his mini-engineering skills and the patient is properly taken care of.

We do have training programmes for doctors too and it would be ideal if a medical doctor would work with a dental practitioner in a co-ordinated way. Until this happens, the dentist who has the case in front of him will have to take charge of it. For a doctor who has seen the light as it were, it is particularly depressing having to work within the western medical system; yet it is possible to make changes even if they are taken in small steps.

PATIENTS

At this time, it is very difficult for a patient. Most of them feel alone and abandoned by the dental and medical professions and with good reason. Your doctor thinks you are a mental case and the dentist does not want you to tell him his job. Both have been doing what they do for years and see no problems. As Dr LD Pankey, one of the greatest dentists of the 20th century, once told me, 'I see dentists make the same mistake for 20 years and call it experience.' Your family may become alienated against you and you are driven into poverty paying the fees for well-meaning, in the main, practitioners of all descriptions doing what they do to you, but the underlying problem remains.

Distance examination

If it is impossible for you to come to us or one of our certified dentists or doctors, then we can act in a supervisory role at a distance. If you ask for one of our information packs and return it to us with the x-rays and scans and other information asked for, we can help point you in the right direction. Without actually seeing you face to face as it were, it is impossible to define an exact treatment plan, but vast experience over the years has taught us what is needed in the majority of cases. Tests for pH levels of urine and saliva can be done at home; even a form of metabolic typing test is available for home use.

224

Results

It is not rocket science after all, more housewives' common sense, metal is metal, infection is infection, and structure is structure; all can be assessed at a distance. It is not perfect though and things can be missed that would be picked up face to face, but it is a damn sight better that rushing round having amalgams removed etc. without the proper protection in place. Patients who come to us after having amalgams and root-treated teeth extracted and are still sick, take the longest time to treat and to recover their health.

Do not expect instant gratification or results. Sometimes, especially with mental or psychological conditions, the results are swift and permanent. At other times, recovery is slower and more gradual. It depends entirely on the patient.

CASE STUDY 31

For example, here is a letter we received from a patient in her 60s one year after we started her treatment. The patient had no specific diagnosed complaint. She wrote,

'If you had asked me six months ago if anything had changed, I would have said no. Since then, however, things have begun to change.

1. I am dreaming again.
I had not associated this with the treatment at first. I used to dream quite a lot, but for the past couple of years this seemed to have stopped. Then a couple of months ago I started dreaming an awful lot, but that has calmed down. Now I dream normally with the happy outcome that my sleep seems a lot more refreshing.

---

2. My short-term memory has returned.
I am not forgetting words so often and when I do forget I remember the words much more quickly than I used to. We went to stay with relatives a couple of months ago and on the last day my sister-in-law said to me, "Last time you came to see us, you kept forgetting words and I was quite worried about you, but all that has changed now."

3. No urticaria this year.
Every year for the last four years when I go outside to do gardening, I come in with at least two large wheals on my torso which I thought were insect bites. Every day I would have new ones and they would be very itchy. Last year, I was so fed up with them that I went to my doctor who referred me to the local hospital. They did skin and blood tests, but said I had urticaria; they could find no cause for it. They said I may have Lupus but this would only be a problem in the future. This year I can garden without any reaction at all. *(G M-H comment: this may have been a reaction to insects, pollen or chemicals but her resistance to whatever it was that caused the urticaria has increased after the dental toxicity factors were properly removed so the symptoms did not return. (Note how useful the medical tests were.)*

4. Healing is much faster.
I cut my little finger tip quite badly with a pair of new secateurs, I nearly sliced it off! I put a dressing and a bandage around it. I did not want

to look at it the following morning, but I had to as the bandage was wet. To my utter astonishment the wound showed signs of healing. I had done the same thing a couple of years ago on another finger and it took months to heal.

5. My throat muscles are working perfectly now. When I was in bed and tired I would try and swallow but sometimes my throat muscles would not respond which was very, very scary. It would take some three or four attempts before my throat would begin to work. Now this seems fine. *(G M-H comment: neurological muscle weaknesses such as this are a common effect of dental toxicity. This patient was fortunate that treatment was done before permanent damage had occurred.)*

6. The amount of saliva has increased.
I always had very little saliva, tears, and nose secretions. Suddenly, one evening my mouth filled with so much saliva that I spent the whole evening swallowing and ended up with a sore throat. I have become accustomed to the increase in saliva and even have had a drip on the end of my nose after heavy exertion.

7. The tiredness has gone.
After the treatment, I felt very tired, even exhausted. This came and went in the months after the treatment. The feeling gradually dissipated and now I have more energy and stamina than ever before.'

227

What is noticeable with this patient is the way the body gradually returned to normal function despite years of being exposed to a variety of dental toxins. It took a while to find homeostasis (balance), but the innate healing capacity was still present.

The roller coaster effect

The last point is very interesting. After the removal of the dental toxins in a controlled way, the patient's body seized the chance of recovering to a proper metabolic state. Whilst these recovery adjustments to the various body systems were underway it took time for the systems to balance out against each other. During this time, the patient experienced what we call the 'roller coaster effect' which is very common after successful treatment. The patient's symptoms get better, then relapse a little, then improve and so on. The 'downs' are not as severe as the original symptoms and become successively less pronounced in duration and intensity as time goes on. Maintaining the supplementation and more vitamin C infusions can shorten or even sometimes eliminate this effect. The roller coaster effect is experienced by about half of our patients.

This was a patient that would be regarded as healthier than average by the medical profession which only serves to illustrates the size of the problem we face. How much healthier, happier could the general population be if treated properly? What a saving in money, both personally and for the state, could be achieved if the population were not chronically poisoned.

Reduce your toxic load

As a patient, knowing where to begin this journey can be quite a perplexing riddle to solve. The first step is to take a personal examination of your lifestyle, habits, medical and dental history. You are actually in control of your life; it may not seem so at present, but no matter what the circumstances are, tiny steps can be made to regain control. It is not always a very comfortable thing to do, but it can and should be done. To quote Rudyard Kipling, 'You are the master of your soul'. As a patient you have to lead as 'clean' a life as possible: no recreational drugs, no tobacco, sensible alcohol consumption, non-toxic personal care (shampoos, deodorants etc.) are simple but excellent ways to start. Searching the internet will give a wide choice of such products.

Food

Try to obtain non-chemical food; eat organic where possible and never touch genetically modified (GM) food at all. The science gradually appearing about the negative effects of GM food is increasing all the time, but still the industry behind GM food is trying to literally force it down our throats. They are trying to remove compulsory labelling of GM ingredients so that the public will have no way of knowing whether food is GM or not. The benefits of GM are entirely for the profits of the industrial giants that created them and nothing to do with any benefit to mankind. The genes inserted into plants are not stable. They can and do move from one part of the DNA complex to another with entirely unpredictable results. We advise you not to touch the stuff.

Grow your own is the best if somewhat impractical solution for most of us, but even simple steps like removing skins or soaking fruit and vegetables in a 3% food-grade hydrogen peroxide solution for a few minutes can reduce the chemical content of conventionally-grown foods. Increasing the antioxidant, mineral and vitamin intake is also a sensible thing to do.

Thought techniques

Positive affirmations written and repeated in combination with visualisation is something anyone can do to help improve personal circumstances. Emotional Freedom Techniques (EFT), Thought Field Therapy (TFT) and the Lightning Process can also be helpful.

Other therapies

Therapies such as lymphatic drainage, homeopathy, herbal, acupuncture, spiritual healing, massage, Bowen, cranial osteopathy, NUCCA atlas adjustment, applied kinesiology, iridology, reflexology, Bach flower remedies, flower essences, urine (in a variety of methods!), and neural therapy are just some of the adjunctive therapies that are available.

We have had patients respond well to these therapies, but mainly after the V-Tox therapy has removed the dental toxins. The therapies seem to encourage the body to find a proper homeodynamic balance.

Other detoxification methods

There are a bewildering variety of detoxification methods available. However, sometimes these methods mobilise the toxins rather than just simply removing them and can make the patient feel worse, so care must be taken when embarking on any detoxification regime. It is not the purpose of this book to comment on or recommend any of the various detoxification methods, but some can be helpful if applied correctly in certain situations. Examples are infrared saunas, enemas, colonic irrigation, skin brushing, oil pulling, oil wrapping, hot and cold showering, Epsom salt baths and so on; the list is a long one. Seeking advice and always beginning slowly are sensible things to do when considering any adjunctive therapy or detoxification method.

Dental assessment

The next step is proper dental and medical assessment of your position. From this a plan can be drawn up to remove the dental toxins and begin the healing process. If this proves to be difficult, we would suggest you contact us for advice. It is not easy being a patient out there under attack, but all is not lost, you need perseverance and discipline to make your way through.

Post dental care reaction

Patients often feel angry and frustrated after recovering from an MCD and seek retribution. This is natural, but by and large nonproductive. Attacking individuals or the 'system' serves little, but produces stress and negative feelings for the patient which are seldom good from a spiritual viewpoint. Legal action may be required to initiate positive changes, but this is best done as a group action rather than as an individual seeking redress or revenge. It is better to lead by example than by preaching about it.

CONCLUSION

There is a web site: *www.toxicdentistryexposed.com* that contains further information including scientific references; this will be constantly updated. We can be contacted through this webite. If you have an MCD, we hope this book has inspired you to search for a solution. If you are a friend or relative of someone who has an MCD, you owe it to them to let them read this book. The knowledge must be spread widely and word of mouth is the best recommendation. The book will not attract mainstream attention as it is subversive to the present models of medical and dental thinking and to the pharmaceutical/ food/agrochemical industries in particular. Since these special interest groups control the media, we expect knowledge of the book to spread through cyberspace person to person. We are coming to the end of our professional lives and we want to pass the baton on to others.

Thank you for being part of this journey.

SUMMARY
- The dental profession is the major contributor to these poisons followed by medical treatments and the industrial complex behind modern society.
- We give training to small groups of dentists and certification can be achieved in our methods.
- The certification process is to protect the patients and help prevent dentists taking shortcuts for increased monetary gain.
- The dentist can aid in the recovery from these MCDs, but it requires commitment from the patient to alter their lifestyle.

- Do not expect instant gratification or results. Recovery is often gradual and can include the roller coaster effect.
- Alternative healing therapies may be applied after the dental toxins have been removed.
- Ideally, the doctor takes charge of the case and co-ordinates the healing. He can send the patient to the dentist for examination (in order to assess the dental toxins), arrange the supplementation, the intravenous infusions and the follow-up care. He can, and should, instruct the dentist to remove the identified toxic problems and make sure that the best interests of the patient are served.
- Many people could lead happier more fulfilling lives if they were not poisoned.
- The saving in money to society would be astronomical and the overall effect on mankind would be enormously positive.

INDEX

Lightning Source UK Ltd.
Milton Keynes UK
UKOW04f1805251014

240628UK00005B/232/P